The Bradley Method®

ASSISTANT COACH'S MANUAL

A guide for expectant couples, and those who support them in labor.

By Susan Bek, AAHCC
with Marjie Hathaway, AAHCC

This manual is dedicated
to all the special people who help support laboring families.

Please Note: In this manual we frequently use the term "husband". We do recognize that some couples are not married. You will notice that we also use the terms "father" and "partner" for the same role. Please apply whatever title you prefer. Also, for the purpose of clarity we most often referred to the coach as "he" and the labor support professional as "she".

Additional support and insight contributions by Coni Sherman, AAHCC, Jay Hathaway, AAHCC, James Hathaway, AAHCC and many others.

The American Academy of Husband-Coached Childbirth® was founded by Robert A. Bradley, MD and Marjie and Jay Hathaway for the purpose of making childbirth education information available. The AAHCC provides lectures, workshops, and national affiliation for Bradley Method® instructors.

For the protection of the public, the terms "Bradley Method", "Husband-Coached Childbirth", and "American Academy of Husband-Coached Childbirth" have been registered. Only those teachers currently affiliated with the AAHCC may teach The Bradley Method®. Ask to see your instructor's current certificate of affiliation.

The Bradley Method® National Headquarters
Box 5224 Sherman Oaks, California 91413
(800) 4-A-BIRTH

www.bradleybirth.com

Teacher's Support Line:
(818) 788-6662

This manual is presented to:

_____

On:

_____

*with our deep gratitude for you agreeing to support us
during our upcoming labor and birth.*

*We look forward to working together through this challenging time
so that we can give this baby and our family
the best possible start.*

_____   _____

Mother   *Coach*

This book contains general information, ideas and techniques which have been successfully used by other families to enhance their birth experiences. Please check with your own health care provider(s) and use your own good judgement in order to determine what information applies to your specific situation and which ideas and techniques are appropriate for you. Every situation is different. We make no guarantees or assurances of any kind to anyone. Only you can make the important decisions you will face during pregnancy, labor, and birth.

The information in this book is presented in the hopes that it will inspire you to seek the best and safest options for you, your baby, and your family.

Note: This book represents the combined experiences of many Bradley® teachers and thousand's of their students' births. It represents parent-to-parent knowledge, not medical advice. For any medical issues consult with your licensed medical team, and make wise, informed choices. It is your birth and your baby, choose wisely. Each birth is unique and special...

Have a Happy Birth-Day!

CONTENTS

PREFACE

WHY COUPLES CHOOSE BRADLEY® CLASSES

The childbirth classes that expectant parents choose have a profound influence on the birth experiences they have. Since every parent wants the best for their baby, they should seek out the best childbirth education possible.

Childbirth classes are not all the same.

Most childbirth classes are short (often only 4 or 6 weeks) and taught in large groups. Couples can feel rushed through a considerable amount of information, and often feel lost in a crowd. Because of the limited amount of time, only a few labor techniques can be taught. Many couples find these techniques ineffective in labor; partly because every woman and every labor is different, and partly because the techniques were barely practiced in class. The Bradley Method® is different.

Bradley® classes don't just teach you why you should have a natural birth, they actually teach you how to do it.

Bradley® classes are taught by certified instructors who are experts in the field of childbirth education. The class series is longer and includes many different labor techniques. Plenty of opportunity is provided to practice the techniques and learn how and when to apply them. Classes are kept small, so couples can get the individual attention they need to feel ready to give birth.

Since an unmedicated birth is usually the best for the baby, Bradley® classes stress natural childbirth as an important goal. Using the techniques taught and practiced in class, over 80% of Bradley®-trained couples are able to give birth without drugs. Women learn what they can do to keep themselves healthy and low risk during pregnancy, while preparing their bodies for the challenges of labor and birth. Special attention is given to the dads in class. Excellent coach's training begins with a study of how they can help their partner avoid unnecessary pain in labor. It continues with numerous simple techniques that can turn any caring partner into a great labor coach. These techniques are safe, effective, and have helped over a quarter million families to have spontaneous, unmedicated births.

Bradley®-trained couples are well prepared for labor and birth.

Couples learn how to plan for the birth experience they want and discuss the importance of building a good relationship with their health care providers. The course also covers information that will help couples to be well-prepared even if a complication arises, the baby is accidentally born in the car, or a cesarean section becomes necessary.

Bradley Method® classes provide comprehensive childbirth education and are the best way a couple can prepare for labor and birth.

HOW TO USE THIS MANUAL

GETTING STARTED

This book is for expectant parents and assistant coaches

This manual is designed to serve two purposes. It is a resource for expectant couples who are interested in arranging for additional support in labor. It is also useful as a guide for anyone who has been invited to provide labor support and take on the role of Assistant Coach.

Most coaches will need someone to assist them during labor.

More and more expectant couples are taking an active role in preparing for labor and birth. As they research childbirth issues and choices, they learn about the many roles and responsibilities that traditionally have been filled by the coach. This leads many couples to consider the idea of arranging for some additional labor support. Most coaches want to be able to focus their attention primarily on the laboring mother. Having an assistant coach present to take care of many of the other details allows the coach to remain relatively undistracted and free to give the laboring woman more of his attention and assistance. This manual is for expectant couples who want to learn more about their options for labor support. It is also an excellent way for an assistant coach to learn about his/her role, and to prepare for the upcoming labor and birth.

This manual can help expectant parents organize and coordinate their plans so that when the time comes everything can go smoothly.

Many couples choose to have an assistant coach, some choose to have more than one. Couples sometimes hire a labor support professional— a person who has been specially trained to assist couples in labor. Occasionally there are older siblings that will be present at the birth. In some instances, couples choose to have the grandparents present. Other family and friends may also become involved. No matter who they choose to have support them in labor, this manual can help organize and coordinate their plans so that when the time comes, everything can go smoothly.

This manual can be useful in any childbirth situation. Couples choosing home births, birth center births or hospital births can all benefit from the kind of support a well-trained assistant coach can offer.

A NOTE TO THE EXPECTANT PARENTS

In order to get the most out of this manual, we recommend that you (the expectant couple) read it first. You should discuss together what you would like to have happen during your upcoming labor and who you would like to have support you. When you ask someone to be an assistant coach, you should already have a clear idea of what you are asking them to do, and what role they will play in your labor. Give them their own copy of this book so that they can read through it and learn all about assistant coaching. They will use and refer to this manual often. It can give them suggestions of how to be more involved, and how to become prepared for the labor.

Parents should read through this manual and then give a copy of it to their assistant coach(es).

You might want to highlight this manual as you read through it, marking anything you particularly want your assistant coach to be aware of or to do for you. Give that copy of the manual to your assistant coach when you are done. Now, as they read it, they will be getting all of the information contained in the manual along with an idea of what you feel is most important.

Assistant coaches need training too. Bradley® instructors can provide that training.

All couples need to take a good childbirth class. We recommend the Bradley Method®. The person or people you choose to support you in labor also need to be prepared. You can attend Bradley® classes as a team, including your assistant coach(es), or you can arrange for a class in assistant coaching from your Bradley® instructor. All Bradley Method® instructors are also certified Labor Support Educators, and can provide training for every member of your support team.

INTRODUCTION

HISTORY OF LABOR SUPPORT

Women were never meant to go through labor and birth alone

From the way the process was designed, it appears that women were never meant to go through labor and birth alone. Since the beginning of time, women have sought out the assistance of their family and friends as well as others from the community, to help them through the challenges and stresses of labor and birth.

During the early 1900's a gradual shift occurred in the United States. Women who, until then had historically given birth at home surrounded by loving, supportive people, were heading straight for the hospital as soon as labor began. As Dr. Bradley, author of the book *Husband-Coached Childbirth* and co-founder of the Bradley Method®, puts it, women were no longer giving birth—they were "being delivered" of their babies.

Unexpectedly, this custom of going to a place where you would be assisted by "trained professionals" did not lessen, but seemed to dramatically increase womens' fear about childbirth. It is no wonder really, the horror stories that were commonly told by the mothers upon their return from the maternity wards were frightening indeed. This, coupled with the mandatory, but unnecessary, separation from the loving support of their family, friends and community, left women to face this frightening challenge alone and unsupported.

As a boy on the farm, Dr. Bradley was fascinated with the birth process.

When Dr. Bradley, an idealistic farm-boy from Kansas, entered medical school in 1944, he was very interested in childbirth. He had observed many animals giving birth on the farm. He knew childbirth was not easy, but that animal mothers seemed to know what they were doing. When left undisturbed, they would work with calm determination and seemed to give birth with a sense of pride and joy. The birth of a new animal had always been very exciting to him. For this reason, he chose obstetrics as his specialty, and looked forward to working in labor and delivery.

What he found there was not at all what he expected. He was horrified to find labor rooms filled with screaming, cursing, suffering women who were heavily drugged, stripped of their clothing, strapped down to a table, and left alone; helpless, humiliated and in pain.

He was even more horrified by the number of deaths that occurred. Most were not deaths from childbirth, but deaths caused by the anesthetics being given to "relieve pain".

Human mothers don't have the same instincts. They must learn to give birth.

He wondered why animal mothers could give birth so peacefully when human mothers did not. He had a theorized that our lack of instinct could be responsible. He wondered if women could be taught how to give birth. If they were, could they enjoy peaceful, natural births too?

Humans are perspiring mammals. Dogs, which pant during labor, do so because they need to cool down. Humans do not naturally behave that way.

In 1947, Dr. Bradley began training women how to give birth. He used observations of other perspiring mammals to develop the techniques and practices he taught. It worked wonderfully. Most of the trained women were able to give birth with dignity and joy, and without any medication whatsoever.

Laboring women are more calm and cooperative when their husband's are present.

Dr. Bradley stayed with these women and coached them through labor and birth. Husbands were occasionally allowed to come into the labor room. They did nothing and said nothing. Yet, when they were in the room, Dr. Bradley observed that the mothers were much more calm and cooperative. When the husbands left the room, the mothers became anxious and tense, and relaxed poorly with contractions.

Dr. Bradley recalls one night after a birth, when the new mother showed him an abundance of exuberant gratitude, kissing and thanking him for all he had done. As he explains in his book *Husband-Coached Childbirth*, "I walked back from this joyful scene to the waiting room and saw the frightened, anxious, distraught face of the man whose love and affection had been shared with this woman to produce this child. It struck me like a sledgehammer. What on earth was this lovely woman kissing me for? I am not the least bit interested in having my patients fall in love with me, but I feel deeply the responsibility, as an obstetrician, to see that the act of bearing a child makes them fall more in love with the father of their baby."

Dr. Bradley is known as "the father of fathers"

After careful consideration, Dr. Bradley realized that, as a coach, he was not doing anything that the father couldn't learn to do. So he introduced husbands as trained labor coaches, putting the emphasis on families working together.

The Bradley Method® *ASSISTANT COACH'S MANUAL*

WHO MAKES THE BEST LABOR COACH?

Using fathers as labor coaches, Dr. Bradley had a 96% unmedicated rate.

"The husband should be the one in constant attendance. Because of his love relationship with his wife, he is far more capable of achieving cooperation and helping her self-control than anyone. We therefore call this approach, 'Husband-Coached Childbirth' " explains Dr. Bradley.

WHAT IF THE FATHER IS UNABLE TO ACT AS COACH?

The coach could be anyone the mother chooses.

There can be many reasons why the father may be unable to act as coach. Among these are: women who choose to be single parents, women whose partners choose not to be involved, men who are serving in the military or unable to be present, men whose religion prevents them from taking this role, etc. In cases such as these, the mother needs to choose someone to act as her coach.

The person the mother chooses to coach her needs to be someone with whom she has a close relationship, and is comfortable. She should know she can trust them and rely on them to stand by her through the many challenges they will face together. They should begin working together during the pregnancy. The coach will need to attend classes with the mother, practice relaxation techniques with her, and give her the daily encouragement and motivation she will need to eat well and exercise regularly. He or she will coach her through labor and birth, and provide assistance and support to the mother for at least the first two weeks after delivery. The coach will most likely be involved for a very long time to come.

CAN MEN REALLY MAKE GOOD LABOR COACHES?

As Dr. Bradley is fond of saying, "A well-trained husband can do more for the comfort and relaxation of his wife than any amount of medication." The key here lies in the training.

Well-trained fathers usually make the best coaches.

Most childbirth classes spend so little time on coach's training that the men end up feeling inadequate and in the way. Men today are expected to act as "Super Coaches" for their partners in labor. But without proper training, they are reduced to useless observers.

Bradley Method® classes offer excellent coach's training.

Some people think that men can't be good coaches, but experience has shown that, with the right training, men who have a loving and caring relationship with their partners make the best coaches. The Bradley Method® classes provide excellent coach's training, and can help turn any caring partner into a great labor coach.

Even Dr. Bradley (who attended over 23,000 births, and developed the highly successful Bradley Method®) felt that each laboring woman's husband could be trained to do a better job of coaching her than he could. Men need only to be willing, well prepared, and supported so they can provide the best labor support possible for thier wives.

Throughout labor, each couple works together laying a strong foundation for their family.

Couples need to keep their families intact as they labor and work through all its challenges, so that the exuberant gratitude displayed by the mother after giving birth is not displaced to some outsider, but directed right where it belongs, to her husband. Working together to give birth brings a couple closer, and nothing makes a new father more proud than when the mother looks into his eyes and exclaims, "I couldn't have done it without you!"

WHAT IS AN ASSISTANT COACH FOR?

Assistant coaches do just what the name implies, they assist the coach.

Being a labor coach is not an easy job. A coach often finds it beneficial to have an assistant to help him with the many tasks and responsibilities he faces during this stressful time. Coaches often feel overwhelmed when they do not have enough hands or enough time to do all of the things they are called on to do during labor.

It is not unusual for a laboring woman to want both her head and her feet rubbed at the same time. Just as the laboring mother insists that her coach must not leave her side, she asks him to go get her a glass of juice. As her contraction begins and he must apply just the right amount of pressure in just the right spot on her back, the phone rings. During the often difficult drive to the hospital or birth center, the coach is expected to time the contractions, rub her back, make sure she stays relaxed, massage away her tension, and talk her through it . . . all while driving the car (safely!) to their destination. At this point he is expected to be calm and polite while they go through the many admitting and prepping procedures. Not every man is able to remain calm while both coaching his wife through powerful contractions that are two minutes apart, and looking up her social security number. Oh, and he also needs to run out to the car and get her bag and her pillow that she, of course, cannot do without. He just better not leave her side while doing it! It takes a man with an amazing bladder to stand by a laboring woman's side offering, her the kind of support and attention she needs for ten hours or longer, without a break to take care of his own needs.

Coaching is a huge job. Every coach should consider having an assistant.

If only he had arranged for someone to assist him. He could have had someone there to rub her feet, get the juice, answer the phone, drive the car, find her social security number, run out to get her bag and her pillow, and take over for him for just a minute while he ran to the bathroom. This person would not replace him as the coach, merely assist him with all the external things, so that he could focus his attention on his most important and demanding job of coaching her through labor and birth.

He may also find it comforting to have someone there who can encourage and support him emotionally, so that he can do his best for his family. Most hospitals and birth centers allow (and some even encourage) couples to have an assistant coach. It is important to check at your birth place to find out their policies.

WHO MAKES A GOOD ASSISTANT COACH?

Many couples select a family member or a close friend to be the assistant coach. With the right training, these people make great assistant coaches. Other couples choose to hire a labor support professional as their assistant coach. Some couples choose to have more than one assistant coach.

The assistant coach must be willing to take direction from the coach, and they must have a calming influence on the mother

The person or people who provide labor support to the family must be willing to do whatever the coach needs done. Their job is far less glamorous than the one of coach (they spend most of their time acting as a errand-runner). It is important that the assistant coach can work well with the coach and doesn't mind taking direction from him. It is also necessary that any assistant coach be a person who has a calming influence on the mother. This is an intimate experience in which to be included. The couple must be completely comfortable with this person.

Choosing someone who will continue to have a close relationship with the family is beneficial. This team will work hard together, and together they will bond with this baby. Assistant coaches form a special bond with the family that can last a lifetime.

WHAT IS A LABOR SUPPORT PROFESSIONAL?

Labor support professionals are knowledgeable about the natural course of labor.

A labor support professional (LSP) is a person whom couples can hire to provide support to them as they labor and give birth. He or she usually has a lot of experience and often is specially trained and certified for this job.

Labor support professionals are also known as Labor Assistants, Doulas, Trained Labor Coaches, Birth Partners, and Labor Companions. These are all basically the same thing. Some of the services they provide may vary. Some offer support during pregnancy and teach childbirth classes. Most support and assist the family during labor, birth and the immediate postpartum period. Some are available for postpartum support to help with anything from housework and meal preparation to instruction on new baby care for the weeks following birth.

See page 100 for information on how to reach The Bradley Method®.

Check with the labor support professionals in your area to see what services they have available. Call the Bradley Method® national headquarters to receive a national directory of Bradley® Certified Childbirth Educators, who are also labor support professionals.

WHY DO COUPLES HIRE LABOR SUPPORT PROFESSIONALS?

Hiring a qualified labor support professional is one way parents can prepare for a positive birth experience. Labor support professionals can act as the assistant coach and provide the reassurance that many couples need. That reassurance can give couples the confidence in themselves and their bodies necessary to accomplish a natural birth.

Couples hire medical professionals (doctors, midwives, nurses, etc.) who watch for any signs of abnormality and handle any complications that may occur. Labor support professionals can act as the expert in normality, helping couples find the most efficient ways to handle their labors and providing the kind of physical and emotional support that can be invaluable to a laboring couple.

Labor support professionals can help a labor to seem more calm and private.

Some couples are concerned about handling labor and birth privately and cannot imagine having an outsider to support them during this intimate time. Most of these couples are planning hospital births, and giving birth in a hospital is anything but private. There are many strangers (medical staff whom they have never met) coming and going throughout labor. A hospital birth is not a private experience anyway. The LSP can remind people to enter the room quietly and help to answer their questions so that the coach can spend more of his time focused on the laboring woman. By limiting the distractions and keeping the couple from being disturbed too often, the LSP can make the labor seem more private than if he or she wasn't there.

Isn't labor support the nurses job?

Some couples mistakenly believe that a nurse will be assigned to them who will teach them whatever they need to know to handle labor, and that he/she will do a lot of the coaching for them. This is not the nurse's job. The nurse usually has several patients he/she is managing at the same time. Nurses are skilled medical professionals who are responsible for monitoring the mother and baby during labor. They spend much of their time on documentation (paperwork) and are responsible for contacting each woman's doctor and carrying out her doctor's orders. They act on behalf of the physician so that he or she does not have to come in until the delivery, if at all possible. The nurses have plenty of work to keep them busy. They do not usually have time to provide the emotional and physical support that many couples need during labor. When couples ask a nurse to help them better handle labor, they most often get medication. Nurses do not have time work with the couple to find more efficient labor positions or more effective coaching techniques. Most nurses have not been trained as labor support professionals. This is a whole different specialty. Couples who want to have additional support in labor need to arrange for it in advance.

Labor support professionals are uniquely qualified to guide couples through the experience of labor and birth. They can help to explain what is going on, reassuring couples when everything is progressing normally, and helping them to recognize the different stages of labor. They are available to answer questions so the couple can make informed decisions and work cooperatively with their medical team. LSP's give the coach any extra "on the job" training that may be necessary as he assists the mother into efficient positions, and uses various natural pain-relieving techniques.

Labor is stressful and exhausting for both the mom and dad-to-be. The encouragement provided by a labor support professional gives couples the strength and confidence to be their best and do what's best for their baby.

"Will you mind taking direction from the coach and doing a lot of the less glamorous jobs?"

The labor support professional you choose should first fit the same general criteria you would have for a family member or friend acting as an assistant coach. It is necessary that they can take direction from the coach and do not intimidate him. They must have a calming influence on the mother and be generally positive and reassuring.

"How many births have you supported? What percentage of those were unmedicated?"

Next, you should check to see that they have plenty of experience with natural childbirth, and specifically with Bradley®-trained couples. It will do you little good if you end up having to convince **them** that everything is all right, and show them how to achieve a natural childbirth.

"What do you feel is your role during our labor?"

It is also important that you feel they are emotionally supportive of you. They should be focused on helping you achieve the birth experience you desire. They should not be trying to heal their own previous bad experience. You are hiring them to support and encourage you through your birth experience, not the other way around.

"Are you certified? What training have you had in this field?"

Check to see if the labor support professional you are considering is certified. All Bradley Method® instructors and some others are certified labor support professionals. Ask to see letters from, or speak with, couples they have previously supported. Verifying their qualifications and checking their references will help you to feel more comfortable with their skills.

"How will we reach you when it's time and what if you are not available?"

It is necessary that any labor support professional you hire be reliable and available when you need them. They generally carry a beeper so you can reach them at any time. Ask them what happens if the labor goes on longer than expected. Find out if they have a back-up LSP they work with in case they become ill or for some reason cannot be available when you need them. How many births have they been hired for and been unable to attend due to personal or other reasons?

"In what ways will you be able to support the coach without replacing him?"

Good labor support professionals seek to empower the family by supporting the coach without replacing him. In situations where they, because of their knowledge and experience, have a suggestion of a position or technique that might be helpful, they teach the coach how to do it for the mother. They might place their hand over his to show him how to better rub her back, but they would not take over and do it for him. This is an important thing to look for when choosing a labor support professional.

"Are you experienced at providing support for the family and not just for the mom?"

This is your birth experience. You (the expectant couple) are building the foundation of your family. You are learning how to work together, learning patience, endurance, and all the other qualities that will make the two of you better parents and prepare you for the challenges and struggles of the future. The job of coach belongs to the Dad (or person of mom's choosing). Even if he makes some mistakes, they are his mistakes to make. He will learn from his mistakes. The family will be strengthened by what he learns. He may want and need support and encouragement, but he must not be replaced. The family needs to struggle together through this challenge. No matter how experienced a labor support professional may be, he/she cannot do as good a job of coaching as the husband can, and it is not his/her place to try. With the help of a good labor support professional he can become an even better coach, but he is the one who loves this mother. He knows her intimately. His encouragement and support mean more to her than an outsiders' can. Together you share the love and commitment for this child. Together, you made this baby, and together you can and should labor to bring it into the world, so together you can face the challenges ahead.

"Is there anything you don't feel comfortable doing as an assistant coach?"

Most labor support professionals do have limitations and personal preferences about what they do and don't do for the couples they support. Perhaps the LSP you are interviewing feels uncomfortable driving couples to their birth place or has a bad back and cannot do anything that would strain her back. Perhaps the LSP would be happy to take pictures for you, but wants to be sure that you understand that she is not a professional photographer. She may not want you to be disappointed if the pictures are not of the quality you might like. Find out if this LSP has any limitations you should know about.

"How much do you charge and what does it include?"

Finally, ask what fee they charge. Good labor support professionals are highly trained people who remain on call for their clients and work very long, hard hours. This is an exhausting and emotional business. They provide an extremely valuable service. Still, compared to what the medical people charge for their services, the labor support professional generally offers her clients an incredible value.

It is recommended that couples who hire a labor support professional give the LSP a copy of this manual, and meet with before the labor to make all the necessary arrangements, and to discuss the things contained in this book.

HIRING YOUR CHILDBIRTH EDUCATOR AS A LABOR SUPPORT PROFESSIONAL

Bradley® instructors are also labor support professionals, and make great assistant coaches.

Hiring your Bradley® instructor to also work as your labor support professional has many unique benefits. Your Bradley® instructor is someone you come to know very well during the last trimester of your pregnancy. She has time to get to know you and your special desires and concerns. She is fully aware of the positions and techniques you have learned and are planning to use in labor. You have many opportunities to observe her skills in supporting and teaching coaches, without replacing them as she leads you in weekly labor rehearsals. You know she has a strong commitment to natural childbirth, and the knowledge and experience you are looking for in an LSP.

Your Bradley® teacher may be the one who educated you, but she is not going to make decisions for you.

A class is a very different environment from a labor room. It is important things in class are taught in generalities. The details of any particular concern or complication that arises during your labor must be discussed with your medical professionals. Much of the information and training you receive in class will be applicable during your labor. If a complication or concern does arise, you need to remember to be flexible and willing to do whatever is necessary to keep the mother and the baby safe. Having a beautiful, natural birth is an important goal, and can have a positive effect on a family which may last a lifetime. However, the health and safety of the mother and baby must come first. If an emergency does occur, crucial decisions affecting their lives and health may need to be made quickly. You should remain flexible and cooperative.

Your Bradley® teacher is someone you can feel comfortable with.

Knowing that your Bradley® teacher will be there to support you during your labor and birth can be very comforting. Expectant mothers often need all the encouragement and support they can get. Expectant fathers are often concerned about remembering all they have learned. Their Bradley® teacher is someone that they know is experienced, knowledgeable, and with whom they have built a good and trusting relationship. Attending classes regularly is still important. These classes provide the opportunities you need to practice together and prepare for the labor and birth. Coaches still need to be well trained. Mothers still need to practice and learn. Having a Bradley® LSP is not an excuse for taking your training less seriously. There is so much to learn in only a little time. Make the most of your time!

Medical professionals and labor support professionals compliment each other wonderfully.

Your labor support professional will not give medical advice. Your medical team is in charge of that. The medical professionals you have chosen are solely responsible for the prediction, diagnosis, and treatment of any complication or risk factor. Your labor support professional does not do vaginal exams, take fetal heart tones, deliver babies or give any medical treatment at all. She can only provide information on natural ways to handle the normal challenges of labor and birth.

Everyone should work toward the same goal; the best and safest birth experience possible for this family.

One of the things you should know in advance, is that your labor support professional cannot answer medical questions. She can discuss with you any natural alternatives she is aware of that have worked for others in the She can act as your consultant on the natural process of birth. She can give you ideas of suggestions she may have and ideas of additional questions to ask your medical professionals. Your LSP may be able to explain any of the medical terminology you don't clearly understand, but she will not make decisions for you, and she cannot confront your medical team. The LSP must be careful to work cooperatively with you and your medical team. If she over-steps their boundaries in any way, the medical professionals may ask her to leave. She has no control over their decisions.

Couples need some time to labor together privately. When the labor picks up, their need for support increases.

Bradley® labor support professionals are happy to talk with you on the phone while you are laboring alone at home. When you get into late first stage labor, and are getting to the point that you need more of their support, they come to assist you. Couples often meet their assistant coach at the hospital or birth center. For a home birth, the Bradley® LSP generally comes after the labor is well-established and your Certified Nurse-Midwife or her Registered Nurse Assistant has arrived.

If you hire your Bradley® instructor as a labor support professional, you will need to schedule a meeting outside of class to discuss her role in your labor and everyone's personal choices. Please see page 61 for more about what you should discuss at that meeting.

ASSISTANT COACHING

SO YOU'VE BEEN ASKED TO BE AN ASSISTANT COACH

Congratulations!

Only special people are asked to be the assistant coach.

Couples only choose to ask special people whom they feel they can count on and work well with to support them in labor. Whether you are a friend or family member who has never done this kind of thing before, or someone who has attended a few births, or you are the most experienced labor support professional, you should feel privileged. It is a very special honor to be asked to be an assistant coach, and it is a rare treat to be able to take part in and witness the miracle of birth. This is going to be a very exciting challenge.

Your Goal

The goal of the assistant coach is to give the laboring couple the support they need to achieve their goals and to help them get their family off to a strong start.

YOUR ROLE AT THIS BIRTH

Assist the coach

The assistant coach frees the coach up so that he can keep his focus on the mother.

Your main responsibility as an assistant coach is to do just as the name implies, **assist** the **coach**. The job of assistant coach is not a glamorous one. You will act as a second pair of hands that will be available to help with whatever the coach needs done. You are the one who will take care of all the background work so that the coach can keep his primary focus on the mother.

Stay positive and enthusiastic

As an assistant coach, you will need to stay positive and enthusiastic. Couples during pregnancy and in labor are very vulnerable to negative influences. Negative attitudes cause the mother to be afraid. Fear causes tension, and tension causes pain. This is a very important point to remember in labor. **Any tension in the mother will cause her pain**. Your help is needed to keep things as calm and peaceful as possible.

Respect this family and their decisions

The assistant coach supports the decisions the parents make.

It is important that you respect this family and their decisions throughout the pregnancy, labor, and birth. They may be making choices that are different from those you would, have, or will. They are responsible parents who are doing things the best way they know how. This is their baby. They have the right to do things their way. As the assistant coach, you have the responsibility to respect their decisions.

PREPARATIONS

Discuss your specific role with the parents

See page 61 for a list of things you should discuss with the parents.

You will need to meet with this couple and discuss the specifics of what they would like you to do. Being familiar with their expectations of you will make it much easier for you to do a good job for them.

Be flexible

As you discuss personal choices and each other's feelings, remember to be flexible. You or the couple may feel differently once the labor begins. Mothers are often concerned about being discrete when thinking about labor, but most will gradually loose their modesty during labor, and by the end of it they do not care about modesty any more. Right now, you may feel unsure about being present during such intimate times, but once in labor and working together with this family, you will probably feel differently.

There may be certain times during the labor when you will need to be present and actively working with the couple. Other times they may need their privacy, and you should step out. Try to stay flexible, and please do not be offended if you are asked to leave for a while. Labor can be a very intimate and private time. Do any background work you can to support the couple while you are out of the room (see page 45 for suggestions of things you could be doing, and stay close at hand ready to assist when the coach needs you).

Pack a bag

Your bag should be packed well in advance of the due date, and kept with you (or in your car) at all times. This way, whenever it is, wherever you are, you'll be ready.

Pack well in advance to avoid additional stress later.

Your bag should include:

❏ Comfortable shoes

❏ Personal toiletries (hairbrush, toothbrush, deodorant, etc.)

❏ Breath freshener

❏ Food to snack on for you and the coach

❏ A sweater (laboring moms often like the room cool)

❏ Watch with a second hand or a stop watch to time contractions

❏ Items to distract and pass the time (i.e. cards, games, books, music, projects)

❏ Phone numbers, and change or a credit card for phone calls

❏ Camera, film, batteries, etc. (if required)

❏ Other items for your comfort, convenience, or entertainment

Make necessary arrangements

Due dates are just an educated guess as to when the baby will come.

Try to make whatever arrangements are necessary so that you can be available whenever you are needed. Normal labors can range anywhere from three hours to three days in length. They can also stop and start several times before the baby is finally born. Due dates are only an estimation. They represent an educated guess as to when the baby will be born. They can be off by two weeks or more in either direction. Research shows that for many women the average length of pregnancy is forty-one and one-seventh weeks,[1] which may be eight or more days after the due date they have been given. This is just an average; every pregnancy is different. Take all this into account as you arrange for time off work, baby-sitting, or whatever is necessary in your situation.

Are there any times when you cannot be available? If so, be sure to let the couple know in advance. You may choose to carry a beeper or phone

---

[1] *Obstetrics & Gynoecolgy Vol. 75, No. 6*

with you at all times. If not, please be sure to let the couple know how to contract you.

BECOME FAMILIAR WITH THE PROCESS OF LABOR AND BIRTH

The stages of labor

You should become familiar with the stages of labor so that you can have a general understanding of how labor progresses. Also see page 67 for more information.

This includes all the labor signs that come and go before the labor begins.

Pre-Labor (sometimes called false labor) - This stage generally involves irregular contractions that often last less than sixty seconds. These are sometimes called natural labor contractions or Braxton-Hicks contractions. It is difficult, if not impossible to distinguish pre-labor from early first stage until it subsides. These contractions will often subside when the mother changes her activity or eats lightly. Pre-labor is common. It may come and go for weeks before the actual labor begins. These "false-alarms" are frustrating, and everyone involved needs to stay patient and reassure the mother that the baby will come when it is the right time. Pre-labor is good practice for all of you.

This is the stage when most mothers are not sure if they are in labor or not.

Early First Stage - This stage generally involves contractions that are ten minutes apart or less, and last forty-five to sixty seconds. They are usually so strong that the mother has to stop and concentrate during her contractions at this point. The labor is just getting established, so it is important for the mother to stay calm. If she becomes too upset, anxious or excited, adrenaline will be released in her body, and can slow or even stop the labor. It can also cause the contractions to become more painful. The mother is generally excited, active, hungry, thirsty and still modest during this stage, which usually lasts many hours, or can come and go for days. When a mother has a very short labor, she spends very little time in this stage, and may skip it all together.

This is the stage when most mothers know they are in labor but they haven't gotten to the hard part yet

First Stage - This stage generally involves contractions that are becoming stronger and more frequent; usually five minutes apart or less, and lasting approximately sixty seconds each. The mother and the labor are settling into a pattern. There is a feeling of certainty that this is labor even though it is likely to be many hours before the birth. It is even possible for the labor to stop for a while, beginning again hours or days later. The mother is generally calm, committed, and usually prefers to keep busy between contractions.

During this stage mothers come to realize why they call it 'hard labor'.

Late First Stage - This stage generally involves contractions that are quite close together, perhaps two to three minutes apart with each contraction lasting sixty seconds or longer. The contractions are often extremely intense during this stage and the mother becomes very serious about what she is doing. She appreciates any encouragement and assistance, but she can not tolerate any disruptions. By this point the mother is loosing her modesty. This is usually a challenging time for the laboring couple. The mother may need a lot of assistance from the coach, and he may need a lot of help from you.

This is a time when labor continues but there is no apparent progress.

Natural Alignment Plateau (N.A.P.) - As many as twenty-five to forty percent of unmedicated women experience a natural alignment plateau during labor. This is a period of time when uterine contractions continue to be intense and frequent, but cervical dilation does not increase. It can be very discouraging to the laboring couple to be working so hard, but not have any progress show in her dilation. The couple needs to be reassured that they are still making progress.

Labor is much more than dilation (opening) of the cervix. The baby may need more time to align itself within the mother's pelvis. The mother's body may need more time to secrete the hormones and enzymes that increase the flexibility of her ligaments and tendons, and soften her cartilage so her pelvis can expand to accommodate the baby. The mother's breasts may need more time to produce the very important immunities she will give the baby immediately after it is born by breastfeeding. The baby may need more time, and more contractions which massage and stimulate it and help prepare it for breathing. This stage may last for hours, but usually ends with very rapid dilation, followed by the urge to push. Even women who are experiencing a N.A.P. at two or three centimeters dilation can dilate to complete and begin pushing within a contraction or two once their body has completed this process.

During this stage, the mother's body shifts from first stage (labor) into second stage (giving birth).

Transition - This stage is commonly marked by confusion as the mother completes the labor and is about to begin second stage (pushing). Mothers are often upset, unsure, and scared. They experience self-doubt. They may have a hard time relaxing, may yell at their coach, and may give up. Mothers can be sweaty, shaky, hot and then cold, nauseous, may vomit, burp, or have cold feet. The contractions may continue hard and close together, double peak, come one on top of another, slow, or even stop. Not every woman has a difficult transition. Some will progress quite smoothly from late first stage into pushing with no transition stage at all. This stage lasts an average of ten to thirty minutes and ends with an urge to push. For more information, see "Understanding Transition" on page 84.

Second Stage - This is the pushing stage. Mothers' contractions change to the expulsive type, and they begin to push with them. At the beginning of second stage, the mother usually gets the urge to push. You and the coach will probably recognize it in one of four ways: 1)The mother may say (or shout), "I have to push!"; 2) The mother may begin grunting or holding her breath and bearing down with contractions; 3) The mother may begin insisting that she feels like she is going to have a bowel movement; or 4) The mother may get to a point that she can no longer relax with contractions, struggling with the contraction until the coach suggests she try to give a little push. If pushing feels much better to her, she is experiencing her urge to push.

Mothers are no longer modest during second stage. They usually appear calm and determined, and are often more alert and talkative between contractions than during late first stage. There are many different pushing positions the mother can choose from. She may decide to use a semi-squatting position, or lie on her side. She might use a hands-and-knees position or one of the other various pushing positions. (The coach's Bradley Method® *Student Workbook* shows and describes many different pushing positions on pages 48-49.) The coach will help her adjust her position between contractions. He may ask you to help him as he makes the adjustments necessary to help her get comfortable in this new position.

The classic position is common but, some women choose to lay on their side, get on their hands and knees or kneel down to push.

In most positions, she will need to pull her legs back (while keeping her elbows up and out) and put her chin on her chest as she rolls up and curves her spine during contractions. She will probably choose to hold her breath for short intervals during pushes. The coach will encourage her to push to the point of comfort, and to hold her breath only as long as she feels comfortable. There are likely to be much longer rest periods between contractions during this stage, which can last only a few minutes, but averages approximately two hours, and can be longer.

As the baby comes down the birth canal, a small amount of the head will begin to show. The baby typically comes two steps forward during contractions, and moves one step back between contractions. At this point some babies come very quickly, but it can be an hour or more from the time you can see a little of the head until the baby is completely born. In some cases, the doctor or midwife may do an episiotomy by taking a pair of scissors and making a small cut in the mothers perineum (the tissue between the vagina and the anus). Many couples choose to try to avoid an episiotomy, and sometimes use warm compresses, massage, and other techniques that can help this tissue stretch better so it won't have to be cut.

This is the time from when the baby is born until the placenta comes out.

Third Stage - The time between when the baby is born and the placenta (or afterbirth) is born is called third stage. Unmedicated babies are usually handed to their mothers as they are evaluated by the medical team. The baby will be wet, and it may be coated with vernix (a cold-cream like substance that protects its skin while inside the water), blood (from the mother) and/or meconium (baby's first bowel movement). It looks both "yucky" and beautiful. The baby will probably open it's eyes, and may make crying or gurgling sounds. If an episiotomy was done, the medical team may need to suction the baby a little to help clear mucous from its nose and throat. When babies are born from an intact mother (one who has not had an episiotomy), they naturally spit out the mucous from their mouth, nose and throat during a process known as the fetal Heimlich maneuver. If an episiotomy was done or a tear occurred during the birth, the doctor or midwife may begin to repair it now. When it is time for the placenta to be born, the mother may feel another urge to push. She will push gently, and the placenta will either come out or be gently lifted out by the doctor or midwife. If you would rather not see the placenta, look at the baby instead. The cord is usually cut by the coach or a member of the medical team at this time.

If this is the first time you have been an assistant coach, you should see a childbirth video in advance. Make arrangements to come to a Bradley® childbirth class with this couple so that you can see a video and practice some labor techniques together. If you are unable to attend a class, you may be able to borrow a video from their Bradley Method® instructor.

The B.E.S.T. way to handle labor

To learn more, please read the article on page 70 and see if you can fill in the questionnaire on page 80.

The coach has been trained to help the mother use Bradley® Energy-Saving Techniques (B.E.S.T.) during labor. These techniques include certain activities that can be very important to the normal progress of labor and help a mother to conserve her energy. They are:

A. **Don't pay attention too soon**

B. **Face the labor calmly**

C. **Go back home if you arrive at the birth place too early**

D. **Use relaxation to handle contractions**

E. **Use normal abdominal breathing during labor**

F. **Walk during labor**

G. **Keep drinking during labor**

H. **Eat if you're hungry**

I. **Sleep if you're sleepy**

J. Stay active as long as possible

K. Try taking a warm bath or shower

L. Avoid taking medication

M. Be aware of natural effective techniques to speed labor

N. Push only when you're ready to push

O. Use positive pushing techniques

P. Be aware of effective pushing positions

Q. Have a happy birth-day!

Some procedures that may be done in labor

Most parents who take Bradley Method® classes are interested in allowing their labors to follow a natural course. They often choose to limit medical interventions, and have very few of the routine procedures often done to medicated moms. Some of the following procedures may be planned during the labor you will attend; others may not. Any or all of them will be done if it becomes necessary and appropriate to do them.

Responsible parents will do whatever is necessary to give their babies the best and safest birth possible.

Every parent wants to end up with a healthy baby and a healthy mother. Since having a natural birth is most often the safest and healthiest for mothers and their babies, parents need to be well-trained and dedicated to having a natural birth. This may mean that they have to work very long and very hard to do what is best for their baby. Your help may make the difference in their being able to accomplish this goal. In some cases, medical intervention is necessary, and can save lives. We encourage parents to remain flexible during their labors, and if intervention becomes appropriate, they will need to compromise their hopes for a beautiful natural birth and do whatever is necessary to end up with a healthy mother and a healthy baby.

Shaving the Pubic Hair—Shaving of the pubic hair is a tradition that began in an era before hygiene became widespread, because mothers would come to the hospital with pubic lice. Since this is not often a concern today, most mothers are not shaved during labor.

Enema—Another old tradition is to give the laboring mother an enema to "clean her out" for the birth. Since it is common for mothers to have several loose bowel movements during early first stage labor, it is usually unnecessary to have an enema. It is sometimes done in cases where the mother is constipated.

Blood Sampling—A standard hospital admitting procedure is to draw a blood sample from the patient to determine the blood type and run a series of tests. If the birth you will be attending will take place in a hospital, you can expect this will be done.

Vaginal Exams—A member of the medical team may insert a gloved hand or finger into the mother's vagina during labor to assess the dilation (opening) and effacement (thinning) of the cervix, and the presentation (position) and station (descent) of the baby. Laboring mothers often find this procedure uncomfortable and need a lot of coaching to help them through it. This information may help to determine if a mother is in labor, and how quickly the labor may be progressing. **Unfortunately, these estimates are not very reliable. They can change quickly or slowly. They do not accurately tell you how much longer it will be before the birth.**

IV—It is possible that the mother could be given intravenous fluids during labor. It is usually not necessary for an unmedicated mother to have an IV. It may become necessary if medication is to be used, a complication arises, the mother is exhausted, or she has become dehydrated. The insertion of the IV is an uncomfortable but brief procedure, and will likely be done between contractions if possible. An IV can be hung on a pole with wheels so the mother can still benefit from walking and using the bathroom often.

Electronic Fetal Monitoring—Most hospital births involve the use of an electronic fetal monitor (EFM)[2]. Most home and birth center births do not use electronic fetal monitoring, but do monitor the baby with either a fetascope[3] or a doptone.[4] Most often, an external fetal monitor[5] is used by attaching two belts around the mother's abdomen or having her put on a special binder (or "girdle") that the monitoring devices can attach to. One of the attachments monitors the baby's heart rate with an ultrasound device. The other, a tocodynamometer[6], monitors the frequency and relative intensity of the contractions. Many parents are concerned with the ultrasound exposure and the lack of mobility caused by the external fetal monitor (because the mother has to stay still while it is in use). For these reasons, many couples ask their medical

---

[2] *An electronic device that monitors and records the fetal heartbeat, as well as the frequency and relative intensity of uterine contractions.*
[3] *A special stethoscope designed to allow the clinician to auscultate (hear) the fetal heartbeat.*
[4] *An ultrasound device that allows the clinician (and/or the parents) to hear an electronic reproduction of the fetal heartbeat.*
[5] *An electronic fetal monitor with probes that are used externally (on the outside of the mother's body). This device uses ultrasound.*
[6] *The part of the external electronic fetal monitor which acts as a pressure gauge. It monitors the frequency.*

professionals to use the monitor only intermittently as long as everything appears normal.

The American College of Obstetricians and Gynecologists (ACOG) and the World Health Organization (WHO) have stated that it may not be necessary to use electronic fetal monitors during normal labors[7]. Recent studies question their value and cite an alarmingly high incidence of false positive readings that, "lead to cesarean sections that are performed without benefit and with the potential for harm".[8] In case of a complication, it may be necessary for the external fetal monitor to be used constantly or it may be replaced with an internal fetal monitor[9]. The internal fetal monitor requires the use of a fetal scalp electrode which is inserted through the vagina and rotated until it punctures the scalp of the baby and is attached. In cases where fetal monitoring is used, the coach and assistant coach should be especially careful to pay attention to the mother's needs. Always look at and encourage the mother, and do not depend on the machine to tell you how strong is the contraction. What may look like a very minor contraction on the monitor may feel like a major contraction to the mother. **Coach the mother and not the machine.**

Amniotomy—Even though the bag of waters is beneficial to the mother and the baby, and plays an important role during labor, sometimes the decision is made to break it artificially. This procedure is known as an Amniotomy. It is usually done by inserting an amnihook (which looks something like a crochet hook with a sharp barb at the end of it) or a special glove that has the barb on it into the mothers vagina and through the cervix to break the amniotic sac.

If baby comes too quickly

If the baby accidentally comes without your medical team being present, there are a few things which should be done. The coach has had some training in his Bradley Method® class to help prepare him for this unlikely possibility. He will most likely want you to open his Bradley Method® *Student Workbook* to the section on Emergency Childbirth (page 102). This will help remind him of what to do and what not to do.

---

[7] *ACOG Practice Bulletin Number 62 May, 2005*
[8] *N Engl J Med 1996; 334:613-8*
[9] *An electronic fetal monitor with probes that are used internally. It does not use ultrasound but it does require the attachment of an electrode that must puncture the fetal scalp. In order for this to be attached, the bag of waters must have already spontaneously ruptured or be artificially ruptured (Amniotomy). The internal monitor may be used with the tocodynamometer (externally) to record the contractions or an internal catheter may be introduced into the uterus to more accurately record the pressure changes that occur as the uterus contracts. Because the internal catheter involves much more risk than the tocodynamometer, it is rarely used.*

Reading the book Emergency Childbirth by Dr. Gregory White will better prepare you for this possibility.

First of all, stay calm. Babies born quickly are notoriously healthy. When it becomes apparent that the baby is about to be born, stop everything else and help the mother. **Call for help as soon as possible**. With clean hands and a clean towel draped over the hands (new babies are wet and very slippery), the coach should just "catch" the baby. Leave the cord alone (let the professionals take care of it properly). Check to be sure that the baby is breathing, and then put the baby at the mother's breast. When the baby nuzzles at the breast, it causes the uterus to contract and helps to expel the placenta (afterbirth) and reduce bleeding. The coach can rub and stimulate the baby if necessary but **no one should attempt to do mouth-to-mouth or any other resuscitation on an infant unless they are trained and certified to do so.** It can be very dangerous.

What to be ready for

As an assistant coach, there are a few things in particular you should be ready for:

1. A lot of hard work - Labors can take a long time. The average length of labor and birth is 15-17 hours. There will be a lot of work to be done during this time. No one said this was going to be easy.

Seeing a birth video in advance will help you become familiar with how laboring mothers behave.

2. Labor noises the mom may make - Be aware that moms often make a lot of noise during labor. She is going to be doing some of the hardest work she has ever done, but it will also be one of the most important things she will ever do. It is worth the effort.

Most mothers should be encouraged to get up and move around to find the best positions for them.

3. Various positions and activities during labor - Walking has been shown to be very helpful during labor. It can help to speed the labor, open the inlet (top) of the pelvis making it easier for the baby to descend, and decrease pain for the mother. She is likely to walk a lot, so bring comfortable shoes. When she gets tired she will need to use the bathroom, and then rest for a while. There will be times when she may be able to sleep for short periods of time. She may also like standing, leaning on walls and furniture, sitting in a reclined position, lying on her side, hands- and-knees position, and sitting on the toilet. She may find it soothing to take a bath (which is usually fine as long as the bag of waters is intact) or taking a shower.

4. Normal discharge in labor - The mother is likely to have a considerable amount of mucous and blood-tinged discharge during labor. She may need to sit on towels or chux pads to protect the furniture. When she gets up, you should change the towel or pad and put down a fresh one so when she and the coach return everything is clean and ready for them. Avoid direct contact with blood, urine, mucous, and amniotic fluid. Any bodily fluid may be able to transmit AIDS.

If the bag of waters is buldging, stand clear. It may burst and get you wet.

5. The bag of waters breaking - The bag of waters (amniotic sac) can contain anywhere from a small amount to approximately one quart of fluid. It can break at any time, but is most likely to break late in labor. When it breaks, it can drizzle out slowly or it can burst and drench everyone in the vicinity. After the water bag breaks, the mother is likely to have frequent gushes of water.

6. Seeing someone you care about in pain - There is a lot of discomfort and pain involved in most labors. Even medicated mothers experience pain during and/or after labor. It can be difficult to watch someone you care about going through pain. Remember that she is doing this for a very important reason; so the baby can have the best possible start in life. Laboring mothers are very vulnerable and impressionable. In her presence you must remain calm and behave as if you are confident. If you begin to feel overwhelmed, try doing something that will be helpful: hold her hand; rub her feet; give her a pep talk; refill her sipper bottle; run errands for the coach; etc. This is not easy, but it is important. Just like marathon runner, when they get tired and it is painful, she needs to hear "You can do it! Great job! Just a little further! I believe in you!". You would never think to discourage someone who was working that hard toward a positive goal. Only positive encouragement is allowed. If you feel overwhelmed and can't be encouraging, you may need to leave the room for a while and collect yourself.

7. The challenge of transition - Transition is often the most challenging stage of labor. It comes between first stage (labor) and second stage (birth). Only one-third of women have a challenging transition. One-third have a mild transition, and one-third have no transition at all (they just move smoothly from first stage into second stage). Mothers who experience a challenging transition often feel out of control, give up, and ask for medication. It is important that you (and everyone) continue to encourage her at this vulnerable time of self-doubt. Keep in mind that transition is relatively short, averaging only ten to thirty minutes. Your encouragement helps to support her best and noblest intentions. Negative comments only feed her fear, cause her tension and increase her pain. Please read "Understanding Transition" on page 84.

8. Some blood loss during and after the birth - There is always some blood loss during childbirth. Spotting during labor is common. There can be some bleeding during second stage, especially if the mother tears or has an episiotomy. Any blood on the baby as it is born is from the mother, not the baby. There is usually what looks like quite a bit of blood loss as the baby is born. Typically, it is mostly water mixed with a little blood, but it still looks bloody. There is often approximately one cup of blood loss as the placenta (afterbirth) is born.

If you don't want to see the placenta, look at the new baby instead.

9. The placenta - The placenta (or afterbirth) can come out anywhere from a few minutes to an hour after the birth. It looks something like liver. It is a fascinating organ that has served an important purpose which is now complete. It was responsible for helping the oxygen and nutrients cross over from the mother's blood into the baby's. It also helped send waste products from the baby back into the mother's system. Some parents are interested and ask to see the placenta. You do not have to look at it if you don't want to. Look at the baby instead.

10. A feeling of exhaustion when it's all over - Assistant coaches work very hard as they participate in a very stressful and emotional event. There is no thrill quite like being present at the birth of a baby. Immediately after the birth, you will probably feel elated and energized. When things calm down, you may begin to become aware of how tired, drained and sore you are. Try to make arrangements in advance so that you will be able to get some rest after the birth. You will need it.

GENERAL JOBS FOR YOU

Be positive and enthusiastic

No matter what is happening, you need to remain positive and enthusiastic. If you have become tired or concerned and need a break, step out of the room for a few minutes. Remember that the medical team's job is to watch for any possible problems. If they are not worried, you don't need to be. Women have been having babies for thousands of years. Everything is likely to go well. Dr. Bradley had a 96.4% unmedicated rate. Nationwide, over 80% of Bradley®-trained couples have spontaneous, unmedicated births. If there is a problem, the family still needs your positive encouragement. One of the most valuable things you can do is to simply smile. It is calm, reassuring, friendly, and it reminds everyone to stay positive.

Maintain a relaxed environment

Any tension causes pain. The better the mother relaxes, the less pain she'll have.

A calm, quiet environment is vital to a laboring family as they work toward their goal of a natural birth. Relaxation is the key to the Bradley Method®. Any tension in the mothers body during labor causes pain. You can help to set up and maintain a relaxed environment. Help to: set up the pillows the way she likes them, dim the lights, adjust the temperature, turn on quiet music, etc. Find out what the mother likes and arrange it.

Keep her sipper bottle filled and ready

The mother needs to keep her body well hydrated during labor. If she becomes dehydrated, she will have a marked decrease in her energy output and her temperature, blood pressure, and pulse rate may all rise. Under normal conditions, laboring mothers are encouraged to drink at least one tall glass of water or juice every hour. Mothers who cannot do this will most likely need to have an I.V. in order to take in that volume of fluid, the coach has been encouraged to give her a sip of water or juice after every contraction in labor. You can help by making sure that her sipper bottle or cup stays filled and ready.

Communicate positively with the medical team

It is very important to keep communications with the medical professionals positive. This is part of the coach's job. He may ask for your assistance. If he does, here are some ways you can/may help:

Upon Arrival at the Birth Place
- ♦ Use first names (they're friendlier).
- ♦ Be polite.
- ♦ Brief them on what's happened so far.
- ♦ Answer questions happily and as completely as possible. Try to answer as many of their questions as you can so that the coach can stay focused on the mother.
- ♦ Give them a copy of this couple's birth plan.

Getting Settled
- ♦ Ask for anything the coach may need (ice chips, a chair, extra pillows, etc.).

♦ Set up the environment she needs (music, dim lights, temperature controlled to her liking, privacy, quiet, relaxed). A positive, relaxing environment helps remind everyone to behave in a positive and relaxed way.

Let Them Know What They Can do to Help
♦ "We would appreciate it if you could . . ."
♦ "It would be helpful if you would . . ."

Offer Sincere Appreciation
♦ "Thank you for . . ."
♦ "We appreciate your help!"
♦ "Thanks!"

Give Them a Positive Reputation To Live Up To
♦ "I know we're in good hands here."
♦ "This is a great hospital, that's why we're here!"
♦ "You're so kind and gentle, you're a great nurse!"

State the Couples Preferences in a Positive Way
♦ "We are looking forward to . . ."
♦ "It is important to them that . . ."
♦ "Please understand, they feel very strongly about . . ."

Protect the mother from being disturbed during contractions in hard labor

No one unexpected should touch or talk to the mother during a contraction.

Mothers in hard labor are extremely sensitive and should not be disturbed during contractions. No one should touch or talk to the laboring woman during a contraction unless she knows in advance that they will be doing so. Mothers most often close their eyes and concentrate deeply while having contractions in hard labor. When an unexpected sound or touch occurs, they can become frightened. Fear causes the production of adrenaline and can cause the labor to slow down or stop. It can also lead to contractions that are ineffective and extremely painful.

The coach has been trained in how to help protect the mother from being disturbed during contractions. He may need you to help him remember to do these things every time someone enters the room during a contraction in hard labor. They are:

- ♦ **Announce who's there**. The mother should not have to open her eyes and turn to see who has come into the room. Even if someone enters very quietly, the mother usually knows they are there. She may wonder who it is and worry about why they are there. This is not what she is supposed to be focused on. To avoid this problem, you or the coach should simply announce who's there when anyone comes in.

- ♦ **Say to them, "Isn't she doing great!"** It helps the mother to hear this kind of praise and it cleverly alerts this person to the fact that we want only positive comments in this room. When you say, "Isn't she doing great!" the other person almost cannot help but say, "yes, she is!"

Most of the time, it is unnecessary to use the "stop sign". It should only be used when needed.

- ♦ If the person approaches the mother quickly and appears to be preparing to touch her in some way, the coach may use **"the stop sign",** a hand gesture that involves gently and politely raising an open hand and suggests stepping back to give the mother a little more room. As he does this he should politely whisper, "one moment please". Whispering seems to be contagious. When one person whispers, everyone around them begins whispering. This is a clever way of politely suggesting that this person wait quietly for the contraction to be over. You could go over, tell them (in a whisper) that the contraction will be over in just a few seconds.

Laboring mothers often need extra verbal support when someone else is in the room.

- ♦ **Give her lots of verbal support**. You and the coach should continue to give her lots of quiet verbal support and encouragement during this contraction. When someone else is in the room watching her, the laboring mother has a harder time relaxing and generally experiences a little more pain. She needs extra verbal support to get her through the contraction.

- ♦ The coach will **complete the contraction with her**. He should not turn his attention away from her until the contraction is completely over and he has done the things he always does for her at the end of a contraction (gives her praise, a sip of water or juice, etc.).

- ♦ Now the coach will say something like, **"Thank you for waiting. How can I help you?"** The medical professionals are often impressed by how polite the coach is and by what an excellent job he is doing. They usually respond to him by saying something like, "I'm fine thank you. I thought you might need me to help you, but I can see that you are doing fine. Let me quickly check a few things and I'll get out of your way."

This positive way of handling things may be more beneficial than you realize. Even well-trained coaches can become intimidated when a medical professional enters the room. They often respond to this by backing off and asking, "how do you think she is doing?" This leaves him open to any response! The medical professional could answer positively or they might suggest some medication. Medication is rarely offered to couples who handle these situations in this positive way.

Now you know what the coach will be trying to do. You work to support him, and keep everything as positive as possible, as together you protect the mother from being disturbed during contractions in hard labor.

Keep records of the contractions

On pages 121-124 in the coach's Bradley Method® *Student Workbook*, there are columns to write down the timing of the contractions in hard labor. He may ask you to keep the record of contractions for him.

Determine the frequency by timing from the beginning of one to the beginning of the next contraction.

To figure out how far apart the contractions are, you should time from the beginning of one contraction to the beginning of the next contraction. This includes all the time from when the contraction begins, through the entire contraction and all the way until the next one starts. This tells you how frequently they are coming.

Determine the duration by timing from the beginning to the end of the contraction.

To determine how long the contractions are lasting, simply time from the beginning of the contraction until it ends. Write down the time that each contraction starts and the time that it ends. This tells you the duration of the contraction.

Make notes on how far apart they are coming and how long they are lasting as well as any other important comments in the Behavior/ Comments column. It can be helpful to know what time she last used the bathroom, how long it's been since she was checked, etc. You could also write down any interesting comments the mother or coach make. People can say some things that seem very special or funny later.

Each of these columns represent one hour. At the end of each hour the coach should evaluate the progress of the labor and consider the questions at the end of the column. This record makes a nice keepsake for the couple, so it should be kept in their book rather than on a separate piece of paper.

Stay in touch with their family and friends

If the parents wish to include specific people in various ways during the labor, you may need to help coordinate. Keep everyone calm and busy.

It is not always the best idea to notify friends and family when the labor begins. Labors often take longer than people expect, and anxious, caring people tend to call to check-in more often than the laboring couple would like. If the family and friends are aware of the labor, it might be best to ask them not to call. Agree to call them every few hours (or whatever length of time seems appropriate) to keep them informed. You should be the one to keep track of when the next call will be made. You may even be asked to make the call.

If you are asked to call and speak with someone about the labor, be sure your comments are all positive and reassuring. Ask the coach what he would like you to say. It is a good idea to say that it will be a long while before the baby comes. Explain to them that these things take time. Let them know that the mother and baby are both doing fine. It may be best for you to call only one person. If there are others who need to be called, have them set up a telephone tree so that you call one person and they spread the word to the others. It will get you off the phone faster and it will give them something to do. But be careful—the story often gets embellished as it travels along.

If the couple chooses to involve selected friends and family members in various ways during the labor, you may be called on to help coordinate everyone's efforts. The coach will tell you what you can do to help in this way. Do everything you can to keep these people calm and busy.

Know when it's time to step in and help

Don't wait to be asked. Step in and do what you can to help.

The general rule is: don't wait to be asked. If you see something that needs to be done, do it. Make sure that the coach is eating regularly. Make sure that the mother always has water or juice and ice chips (if desired) available. Observe the kind of coaching that the mother needs during contractions so that when the coach needs to run to the bathroom or take a break to eat something, you can step in. Answer the phone when it rings. Wash the dishes, run the laundry, there is no end to the tasks that you may be able to take over so that this mother and coach can focus their energy on the labor.

Know when it's time to step back

There will be times when the couple needs their privacy. If you are asked to leave the room, please do not be offended. They may have asked you to avoid being present during vaginal exams or other procedures. If so, do not wait to be asked to leave, excuse yourself when it is appropriate. If they encourage you to stay, you will know they have changed their minds; if not, you will know it's time to step out. If she has a difficult time relaxing and staying calm when you are in the room, step out for a while. This may be one of the times she needs some privacy. In general, if you are not doing something helpful in the room, step out. Mothers do not like being stared at. Labor is not a spectator sport, it is a team event

Take direction from the coach

Let the coach know that you don't mind his asking for your assistance.

The coach will need a lot of help from you. A prerequisite for this job is that you be able to take directions from the coach. Let him know that you don't mind his asking for your assistance. Offer to do the things you think he needs. Do not get in his way. Do not try to replace him, even if you have more experience than he does. You are the assistant, he is the coach. Let him be the one who calls the shots. Let him do the talking. Put him in the spotlight. If she likes having someone near her face or in front of her, that should be his place. You do more of the "behind-the-scenes" jobs so that he can focus his attention on her. Always look to empower this family; this is a very important part of your job. You will know you have done your job well, if when it's all over, the mother looks up at her coach and tells *him*, "You were great! I couldn't have done it without you!" She will thank you too, but the majority of adoration and appreciation that a mother feels for the help she receives during labor should be directed at her coach.

Look to empower this family

The majority of adoration and appreciation a mother feels for the help she receives in labor should be directed at her husband.

This is their birth experience. These parents have the opportunity to work together through this challenging time and strengthen their relationship. They will need this strength as they face all the daily challenges ahead. You can help to empower this family by always looking to support the coach without ever trying to replace him. Sometimes, because of experience or just a knack for nurturing and supporting laboring women, the assistant coach can do an incredibly great job of coaching and is tempted to take over. This is not your place. The assistant coach should never get between the mother and her coach. Be aware that coach's are sometimes intimidated and will back off when someone else tries to lead. Be careful! Don't look so good that you make the coach look bad. If you have any thoughts or ideas that might be helpful, suggest them to him so he can try them.

Be willing to get by on little thanks

When this is over, you are going to deserve a lot of credit for all you will have done! The mother is going to be thankful for your help. However, if you have done a good job of staying in the background, and supporting the coach by doing a lot of the less obvious jobs, she will never even know just how important you were. That's fine. That's the way it should be. The most important thing is that this family gets off to a great start. You can be proud of yourself and know that you played a major role in the birth of a precious baby and the beginning of a strong, healthy family.

While supporting couples in labor, many people say to themselves, "this is such hard and emotionally challenging work!" Still, every baby deserves to have the best and safest beginning, and every family needs to get off to a strong start. It's when you see the new parents staring lovingly into their new baby's eyes that you'll realize that the fringe benefits are what make it all worth it.

Redirect her praise; the new parents get all the glory

Redirect praise to the mother, father and the family.

When the mother expresses her appreciation, thank her, and then redirect her praise, and give the coach the credit. "He was wonderful, wasn't he! He deserves the credit, he did all the hard work." Redirect praise toward the mother too, "You did such a wonderful job! I can't believe how strong and committed you are! You are absolutely amazing!" Give plenty of praise to the parents together, "You two make such a great team. This baby is so lucky to have you two for his/her parents! I'm so proud of you both! You have a beautiful family!" Take very little of the credit yourself. You are going to step aside now and let this family stand on their own. Together they will face the daily challenges ahead. They need to be made aware of how strong they are together. They are building the foundation for their family. It needs to be built up and made as strong as possible. Taking too much of the credit would diminish their feeling of strength and their ability to stand strong on their own. Stand back and take a good look at that beautiful new family. There's your thanks; who needs glory?

SOME WORDS OF CAUTION

Be careful; don't exhaust yourself

Take breaks when you need them, this job can be exhausting.

It is easy to get excited and exhaust yourself while supporting a couple in labor. You may need to take a break, sit and rest, or take a nap. Perhaps you could trade off with the coach if the labor is a long one. Be careful that you protect your back and respect your own physical limitations. It can be very physically challenging to do this kind of work. It may be your job to see that the coach eats regularly, but be sure that you do too. Most women are disturbed by the smell of food late in labor. You and the coach may need to trade-off helping the mother and stepping out to eat. It is a good idea for both of you to brush your teeth or do something to freshen your breath after eating and before returning to work with the mother.

Do not take any chances

This couple should be in touch with their medical professionals during labor. They will need to call them once the labor becomes well established and/or when the bag of waters breaks. If there are any possible danger signs or any concerns whatsoever, they should check with their medical professionals immediately. Couples can ask their doctor or midwife for a list of danger signs to watch out for.

WAYS THE ASSISTANT COACH MIGHT BE HELPFUL

Every coach and every labor is different. This section lists many ideas of ways you might be helpful. Take your cues from the coach; he will let you know what he does and does not want you to help with.

At home - early labor

The following are some ideas of how you might be helpful during this stage:

This stage generally lasts many hours.

♦ Set-up a peaceful environment.

♦ Handle phone calls.

♦ Wash the dishes.

♦ Prepare food.

♦ Keep her sipper bottle (or glass) filled.

♦ Make sure the car has a full tank of gas.

- Run to the market if necessary.
- Be alert, do what needs to be done (i.e. feed the dog, pick up the kids, run the laundry, scrub the bathroom, etc.).
- Prepare for the Birth-Day party.
- Gather last minute things.
- Change the bed and leave the house clean so it will be nice for the new parents to come home to.

If moving to the birth place

The following are some ideas of how you might be helpful at this point:

If the couple is planning a home birth, you will probably not change locations.

- Prepare the car - place towels or chux pads on the seat where the mother will be sitting, have pillows available for her to use, place a full sipper bottle where she can easily reach it, place a bucket beside her seat (in case she vomits). Other things that belong in the car include: mom's bags, the coach's bag, your bag, the mom's ID, her insurance card (if necessary), a copy of their pre-admittance papers, copies of their birth plan, and any food or drink they are bringing.

A small percentage of home birth couples are transferred to the hospital because of a complication or as a precaution.

- Drive the car if you're asked - See page 120 in their Bradley Method® *Student Workbook*. It should have directions and a map of how to get there. Drive slowly, carefully, follow all traffic laws, and pay attention to your driving, not her laboring. It is very important to get this family safely where they are going. You may have to slow down or stop for contractions.

- Carry in the bags - The coach will help to get the mother inside; assist him if necessary. Your job is to bring in whatever supplies they need from the car. First bring whatever comfort items the mother needs right away (i.e. her sipper bottle, pillows, relaxing music, etc.). The drive and change of location is very disrupting to the labor and may increase her pain. It is very important to set-up a relaxing environment and get her settled as quickly as possible. Laboring mothers tend to move very slowly. You may be able to go ahead of them to her room and get it set up before she comes in. This can be very helpful!

- Help to get her registered - Couples are encouraged to pre-register at the hospital or birth center they will go to in labor, or are using as a back-up. They should keep a copy of their pre-

The Bradley Method® ASSISTANT COACH'S MANUAL

registration forms just in case they are lost. You should know where these copies are and get them out if necessary. There are usually more forms to fill in, and lots of questions to be answered when you arrive. Since the mother and coach will be busy handling the labor and its frequent, strong contractions, you may need to help. Get out her ID so you can answer questions about her driver's license number, social security number, insurance plan information, etc. Be very polite and answer any questions you can. For answers to questions you don't know, wait until the coach has helped the mother through her contraction, and quickly ask him. This process can be frustrating because the coach has very little time during which he can pay attention to these things. Your work to keep things calm and the distractions brief will be helpful for both the couple in labor and the medical team.

♦ Write down the names of the nurses - record anything positive that people do. This information can be helpful when writing thank you notes later.

Active labor

The following are some ideas of how you might be helpful during this stage:

This stage averages two to five hours, but can go longer in some labors.

♦ Be sure the coach is eating and drinking regularly.

♦ Be friendly and speak softly as people come in. Say, "Isn't she doing great!"

♦ Handle the telephone - update the family regularly. Say, "These things take time".

♦ Praise and reassure her - she needs to hear it.

♦ Rub her feet, or hold and stroke her hand.

♦ When she gets up, replace the soiled pad with a clean one so that when she returns all is ready for her.

♦ Get cool wash cloths.

♦ Keep her sipper bottle filled.

♦ Take pictures of the couple working together.

♦ Follow the coach's instructions.

♦ Rub the coach's shoulders.

♦ Take over if he needs a bathroom break.

♦ Keep track of contractions, positions, bathroom, etc.

Transition

The following are some ideas of how you might be helpful during this stage:

This stage averages only ten to thirty minutes.

- ◆ Stay positive and enthusiastic.
- ◆ Encourage her, cheer her on.
- ◆ Assist in any way you can.
- ◆ Don't get offended if she snaps at you.
- ◆ Stay calm and confident.
- ◆ Support and encourage the coach.
- ◆ Take one contraction at a time.
- ◆ Be ready for a change.
- ◆ Watch for the urge to push.
- ◆ Keep their friends and family calm.
- ◆ Remind medical people to come in slowly and quietly.
- ◆ Tell everyone who comes in, "Isn't she doing great!".

Second stage - pushing

The following are some ideas of how you might be helpful during this stage:

This stage averages two hours.

- ◆ Get ice chips for her.
- ◆ Bring her a cool cloth.
- ◆ Assist with her position if necessary.
- ◆ Be encouraging - Smile!
- ◆ Be willing to step out if asked.
- ◆ Encourage her to "open up, push down and out".
- ◆ Remind the coach to be sure she brings her knees back, keeps her elbows up and out, and puts her chin on her chest if she's in the classic (semi-squatting) position.
- ◆ Remind her to relax between contractions.
- ◆ Take pictures.
- ◆ Fan the mom (use this manual or a piece of cardboard if nothing else is available).
- ◆ Stay out of the way of the medical people and equipment
- ◆ Don't touch anything that is sterile or draped with cloth.
- ◆ Don't announce the sex of the baby - let the parents look when they are ready.
- ◆ Notice how alert the baby is when it's born.
- ◆ Look in the baby's eyes.

After the baby is born

The following are some ideas of how you might be helpful at this point:

- ◆ Respect family bonding.
- ◆ Take pictures.
- ◆ If you're a member of the family or a friend, hold and touch the baby when it is your turn. This is why you did all this. This is a very important person in your life.
- ◆ Notice how the baby looks and smells, and what it sounds like.
- ◆ Help collect their belongings.
- ◆ Get food for everyone.
- ◆ When you have the chance, send flowers to the mother. She deserves them.
- ◆ Go to their house - clean, market, run laundry.
- ◆ Write a letter to the baby about what it was like to be present at his/ her birth.

If something goes wrong

The following are some ideas of how you might be helpful if something goes wrong:

Look to the medical professionals to guide you through any complication. That is what they specialize in.

- ◆ Stay calm and positive.
- ◆ Look for the good things - focus on them.
- ◆ Assist in any way you can.
- ◆ If the mother and baby must be separated, the coach will go with one and you will stay with the other.
- ◆ Trust that they have selected a good medical team. They will do everything they can to help the mother and the baby.
- ◆ Step out if you need to.
- ◆ Call their Bradley® teacher for support.

For more detailed suggestions of ways you could be helpful, see page 92.

WHAT ASSISTANT COACHES SHOULD BE CAREFUL NOT TO DO

♦ Don't get between the mother and coach. Let him do the more important jobs. Always look to empower this family.

♦ Don't stand and stare. Labor is not a spectator sport, it's a team event.

♦ Don't show negative concerns to the mother. Always stay positive. The medical team will step in if there is a problem.

♦ Don't announce the sex of the baby when it's born. Let the mother look for herself when she is ready.

♦ Don't call or announce the birth to family and friends unless the coach asks you to. He has earned the privilege of making those calls.

A NOTE TO THE COACH

Your assistant coach(s) want to help. Don't hesitate to ask for their assistance. Feel free to ask them to step out if necessary. They'll understand. Delegate whatever you can. The mother and baby are your first priority.

SPECIAL ROLES FOR SPECIAL PEOPLE

GRANDPARENTS WHO ARE INVITED TO ATTEND A BIRTH

It is a very special honor to be invited to take part in welcoming your new grandchild into the world. Congratulations! Your son or daughter and their partner must feel comfortable with you and have a good relationship with you or they would not be offering you this opportunity.

It is a very special privilege to be invited to help bring your grandchild into the world.

What you are now preparing to do is a special privilege with lots of wonderful benefits, but you will have a special challenge too. There can be nothing else like witnessing the birth of a baby. This is a very special and important baby, too. It is your grandchild. As you go through the long wait for labor to begin, as you experience the nervous anticipation and the fearful concerns that only the grandparents feel (because it is their children who are going through this experience), as you feel the mom's pain and wish you could lessen it for her, keep in mind and look forward to that first moment when you will be able to look into this baby's eyes. Look forward to the time when it is your turn to hold and rock and cuddle and love this bundle of joy. The challenge and struggle of the labor will all have been worth it.

Do everything you can in advance to prepare for this challenge.

We recommend you go through all the information in this book and prepare for your role in this labor. The same information applies, but we would like to add one thing. Your reassurance and praise is very powerful. Because you are their parents, your approval is more important than most people's. Your remaining calm and positive is extremely important. You may find that you have a very soothing and reassuring influence on this couple which has a direct effect on the pain the mother feels during labor. Your presence and reassurance may well lessen the pain for her. Please don't be offended if you are asked to step out and allow them some privacy at times. Just be ready to go back in when you're called to soothe and reassure them again.

This couple may not choose to do things the way you did them, but this is their baby. They are taking responsibility and doing the best job they can do. Be careful not to let any of your concerns show, and never allow yourself to criticize them during labor. Just as you may have the wonderful power to lessen her pain, you also have the power to increase it and even add to her discomfort by upsetting her. To help avoid feeling overwhelmed, keep busy. If you are not needed in the room with the laboring couple, step out and do something else (wash the dishes, prepare some food, read a book, watch television, etc.).

New mothers and fathers need a lot of support and a little privacy too. After the birth you can take on the role of grandparenting, but don't forget your more important roles of parenting. New mothers need to be taken care of for a while so they can have time to adjust and become good mothers themselves. New father's need a lot of support too. Do what you can to be available and to be supportive.

THOSE WHO ARE ASKED TO SUPPORT CHILDREN WHO WILL BE PRESENT AT A BIRTH

Many families now are choosing to involve their older children and allow them to be present at the birth of their sibling. These families must do a lot of extra work to prepare for the birth. They need to prepare their children and arrange for the special support they will need during the labor.

The book _Children at Birth_ by Marjie and Jay Hathaway is an excellent resource. The assistant coaches training provided in this manual will be important and useful to you, but as the person who will support this child or these children, you will play a special role and should do some extra work to prepare.

❖   ❖   ❖

Prepare by discussing your role with the parents and completing the following information (if you will be caring for more than one child, use additional paper):

Child's name:_____

What time does he/she normally wake up in the morning?:_____

What is their usual "wake-up routine"?:_____

_____

_____

_____

Does he/she take a nap during the day? ❏ If so, when and for how long?:_____

_____

What is his/her normal "naptime routine"?:_____

_____

_____

When does he/she normally go to sleep at night?:_____

What is his/her normal "bedtime routine"?:_____

_____

_____

_____

When is he/she used to eating and what does he/she like to eat:

BREAKFAST	LUNCH	DINNER
_____	_____	_____
_____	_____	_____
_____	_____	_____
_____	_____	_____
_____	_____	_____
_____	_____	_____
_____	_____	_____

Usual time: _____   Usual time: _____   Usual time: _____

Does he/she snack during the day? ❑ If so what does he/she like to eat for a snack?:_____

_____

What inside activities would he/she enjoy doing while you're in labor at home?:_____

_____

_____

What outside activities would he/she enjoy doing while you are in labor?:_____

_____

_____

_____

Note: Never take the child anywhere without checking with the parents first.

What quiet activities would he/she enjoy while at your birth place (if other than home)?:_____

_____

_____

_____

Are there any things that he/she is not allowed to do or eat that I should be aware of, if so, what?:_____

_____

What is his/her normal schedule for school, activities, etc.?:_____

_____

_____

_____

_____

What is the address and phone nuber of his/her school, (if applicable)?:_____

_____

Are there any parts of the labor or birth that they particularly want to be present for?:_____

_____

_____

Are there any parts of the labor or birth that you particularly do not want him/her there for?:_____

_____

_____

If he/she is asleep when the baby is coming, do you want me to wake him/her, if so, what can I do to help him/her wake up without upsetting him/her?:_____

_____

For how long after the birth should I be prepared to take care of him/her?:_____

_____

Is there anything else that would be helpful for me to know, if so, what?:_____

_____

_____

❖   ❖   ❖

A bag should be packed for the child in advance of the labor. Work together with the parents to prepare a bag for the child. If there is more than one child, they should each have their own bag. Suggestions of what they might contain include:

❑ **Snacks**

❑ **Quiet activities like: games, toys, books, etc.**

❑ **Drawing supplies: paper, pens, crayons, etc.**

❑ **Comfort items such as a teddy bear**

❑ **Sleeping bag or favorite blanket and a pillow**

❑ **A jacket or sweater**

❑ **A change of clothes**

❏ any toiletries they may need (i.e. hair brush, tooth brush, etc.)

❏ disposable camera or other equipment (if desired)

❏ change for vending machines (if desired)

❏ new, wrapped gifts (just small, inexpensive, quiet things that can be given to him/her for fun when they are bored)

❏ a gift from the child to give to the new baby

It is the parent's job to prepare the child(ren) but it is best if you can be present at the sibling preparation class or at least one of the family's discussions about the upcoming labor and birth.

The children need to be well-prepared. They should be comfortable with the idea that mommy will be working very hard, that she may make a lot of noises and that she may take her clothes off. Children need to understand that labor can be long and boring. They should be aware that eventually she will start pushing and that it will be very hard work for her. They should be prepared for the blood, the pain, and the placenta as well as for the wonder of watching a baby born.

The older the child, the more preparation they may need. Young children are not usually as upset by blood, pain and nudity as older people are.

A good way to prepare children is to share the pictures and stories in the book *Children At Birth* and to show them the video *Children At Birth*. You may be able to arrange for your Bradley® teacher to provide a special class for children who will be present at a birth. She may show them the video at that class. If not, you might ask to borrow the video from her. You might consider buying the video. It can be very helpful for children to view the video at their own pace, turning it on or off whenever they feel like it. They may want to watch it many times and discuss things with you. The book and the video are both available from the Bradley Method®. See page 100 for further information.

It can be helpful if they have certain jobs during labor and birth. Some ideas of jobs for children are:

♦ Make a cake.

♦ Squeeze orange juice.

♦ Massage Mommy's feet with lotion.

♦ Call Grandma every hour.

♦ Draw a birthday card for the baby.

♦ Put up birthday decorations and prepare for a party.

♦ Encourage Mommy, by saying, "You can do it! You can do it!"

♦ Bring Daddy a snack.

♦ Refill Mommy's sipper bottle.

♦ Take pictures of the birth. We recommend either using a digital camera with lots of memory, telling the child to wait until they can see the baby's nose, then let them take as many pictures of whatever they want to. These pictures are precious. Some children can use an entire roll of film on a quarter-sized amount of baby's head showing. These pictures are not very discrete or interesting later. That's why they should wait to see a nose first.

♦ Have a towel or blanket ready for the new baby, who will be born wet.

♦ Rock the baby when it's your turn. Little ones can be allowed to hold the baby if they are sitting in the middle of the bed, where it would not be a problem if they accidentally dropped it. Be careful.

Consider, in advance, what you can do to help keep the child(ren) entertained.

Part of your job is to be sure that they are fed at regular times with the foods they are used to. Do not give them "treats" unless okayed by the parents. The last thing you will need is to deal with bored, nervous kids on a sugar high. You should also be sure they get to rest when they normally would. You will need to entertain them and should take them for short walks, trips to the park or just into another room if the parents prefer. Be sure you never take the children away without consulting the parents first. It can be very hard to know when the baby will be born, and the fear that the children could miss it will increase anxiety and pain for the mother.

If the child needs you elsewhere, you will have to miss the birth.

You must remain willing to take the children out at any time they or their parents request it. You must be willing to miss the birth if that becomes necessary. Your job is to take care of the children first. Witnessing the birth is secondary.

Some parents choose not to have older children present for the birth, but have them come into the room immediately afterwards. This is a good option for some families. The sooner these children are introduced to each other the better, but we do suggest that the messy parts of the mother be covered with a sheet or blanket before the child comes in. Children who are present for the labor and birth and saw how the mess got there are usually fine with it. It is different for children who were not there.

Take lots of pictures, they make great keepsakes.

Be sure you take pictures of the child(ren) as they wait for the birth of their sibling. It is especially wonderful when the child's support person puts these pictures as well as any pictures the child takes, and arranges them in a photo album. The child's own description of the picture makes a great caption!

PHOTOGRAPHING A BIRTH

Couples who want pictures of the birth need to have someone assigned to this task.

The person who photographs the birth also plays a special role. The section of this manual on assistant coaching will be beneficial for you in preparing for this labor. There are a few additional things you should consider and prepare for in advance.

It is important to meet with this couple and discuss what kind of pictures they would like. Will you be using their equipment or your own? Whatever equipment you use, be sure to practice with it ahead of time. If you will be taking still pictures, practice by taking a whole role of pictures and having them developed so you can see the results. If you will be video taping the birth, practice by taking some footage of the expectant couple at home preparing for the birth of their baby. Using a simple camera is usually best. If the camera is too complicated, you may end up with pictures or video tapes that are no good. The birth of a baby is something that cannot be repeated, because the camera wasn't working. Be sure you have plenty of batteries and film or videotape. Pack-up the equipment in advance, and be responsible for it

Some hospitals have strict rules about photography, check this out in advance.

The parents need to make arrangements with their medical professionals in advance. Some people are uncomfortable when they are being photographed. Some birth places have strict rules about photography in their facility. This all needs to be worked out in advance.

Take most pictures from a discreet angle. The mom may not be modest during the labor, but she will be later.

Many parents choose to have their birth videotaped so that they can see it again later. Often, parents will show the video to the child when they get older. There are some special concerns you should consider if you are going to video tape a birth. Labor rooms are often fairly small. It may be difficult for you to move around well during the birth. You might want to set up a tripod or stand in an out-of-the-way part of the room. Look for the side angle; it is the most discrete. Be careful not to use up too much of the tape before the birth. There will be a lot of things to videotape after the birth too. Carefully frame your picture. Avoid views that are unnecessarily graphic. Avoid crotch-shots after the birth. Rarely does anyone want to see an episiotomy repaired. Focus on the family.

Discuss in advance what they would like to have pictures or video of. There are no guarantees that you will be able to get all the shots you plan to. Some suggestions include:

- ❏ The couple working together during labor.
- ❏ The mothers beautiful round belly.
- ❏ The couple walking around.
- ❏ Pictures of their faces as they work together.
- ❏ Pictures of them holding hands.
- ❏ Daddy's hand on her belly.
- ❏ Daddy talking to her belly.
- ❏ Mommy gently rubbing her belly.
- ❏ The baby's room.
- ❏ Each member of the medical team helping and supporting the couple in labor.
- ❏ The assistant coach washing the dishes, taking out the trash, carrying the bags, and all the other things they will be doing.
- ❏ The family waiting in another room.
- ❏ Any special gifts people have made or brought for the baby.
- ❏ Discrete pushing pictures (pictures taken from the side angle are usually discrete).
- ❏ Mommy's face as she works hard pushing.
- ❏ Daddy encouraging her as she rests between contractions.
- ❏ The doctor or midwife getting ready to "catch".
- ❏ The excitement on the faces of the family as the time of birth nears.
- ❏ A few pictures of the baby's head as it begins to show and then comes out. The parents may want you to take them even if they may throw them away. They will never have another chance to see this.
- ❏ Mommy and Daddy's faces as the baby is born.
- ❏ The first time they look into the baby's eyes.
- ❏ Baby breathing and stretching.
- ❏ Baby placed on Mommy's breast.
- ❏ Daddy touching and getting acquainted.
- ❏ Mommy cuddling and kissing baby.
- ❏ Mommy kissing and thanking daddy.

❏ Doctor or midwife congratulating family.

❏ Mommy and/or Daddy holding a precious little hand.

❏ Baby looking around.

❏ Mommy nursing baby.

❏ Daddy cutting cord.

❏ Placenta after it's born. (This is another one of those "you might want to see it later" shots that may end up in the trash, but you may want to take it "just-in-case".)

❏ Daddy holding the baby for the first time.

❏ Baby being weighed and measured.

❏ Baby being welcomed by other family members.

❏ The relieved look on the faces of everyone in the other room when daddy announces the birth of the baby.

❏ Daddy on the phone announcing the birth.

❏ Mommy back in bed, all cleaned up, holding and nursing the baby.

Have the parents list others that are important to them:

_____

_____

_____

_____

_____

Do not show the pictures to anyone until the mom and dad have seen them.

Parents need to be specific about what they want from the photographer, but must also remain flexible. Things can happen fast and you will not get every picture you wanted. You will probably get several you didn't plan for that end up being very special too.

It is very nice when the photographer has the pictures developed and arranges them in a photo album for the parents. It is best to keep any indiscreet pictures separate because the parents may want to keep them private. It is hard to know what the parents will and what they won't want to share with others, so do not show any of the pictures to anyone until the parents have a chance to see them.

REFERENCE INFORMATION

IMPORTANT DETAILS ABOUT THIS BIRTH

These questions can be used as a guideline for the meeting(s) expectant couples have with their assistant coach(es) as they work out the details and plan for this labor and birth. If you are a friend or family member that has been asked to be the Assistant Coach, you may not need to have as much detailed information. Please adapt these questions to your situation and include any information that you need.

Note: The information that you may need to refer to quickly has been placed on the front cover of this manual. Begin by completing the information found there, then continue with the following information.

YOUR BIRTH PLAN

Have you written a birth plan?:_____

How would you like this birth to go; what is your target birth experience?:_____

_____

_____

_____

_____

Have you discussed the fact that you will be having an assistant coach with your medical team?: ☐

Have you cleared it with your birth place (if necessary)?: ☐

MY ROLE AT YOUR BIRTH

What role do you see me playing in your birth experience?:_____

_____

_____

_____

Coach: specifically, what jobs do you see me doing for you in labor? (For ideas of ways the assistant coach can be helpful, see page 45.):_____

_____

_____

_____

When do you think you would like me to arrive?:_____

Do you think you'll want me in or out of the room:

     during vaginal exams?: ❑ In ❑ Out

     while you're in the bathroom?: ❑ In ❑ Out

     when the doctor or midwife is talking to you?: ❑ In ❑ Out

     during the birth?: ❑ In ❑ Out

     if a transfer is necessary? (from home to hospital or from LDR to reg. labor/delivery): ❑ In ❑ Out

     if a cesarean becomes necessary?: ❑ In ❑ Out

       who would go with the baby?: _____

       who would stay with mom?: _____

Do you want me to take any pictures?: ❑ Yes ❑ No If so:

     what equipment should I use?:_____

     how do you operate the equipment?:_____

     who will prepare and bring the equipment and supplies?:_____

    (See Photographing a Birth page 58 and discuss what they do and don't want pictures of.)

Are you packed?: ❑ Yes ❑ No

What coaching aids are you bringing?:_____

_____

What, if anything should I bring for you?:_____

_____

THE WELCOMING COMMITTEE

Will your older child (children) be present at the birth? (if applicable): ❑ Yes ❑ No

If so, who will be their care-giver?:_____

In what ways can we involve them in the labor and birth?:_____

_____

_____

_____

Will any other friends or family members be present during the labor and/or birth?: ❑ Yes ❑ No

If so, who:

Name	Phone #	Alt. Phone/Pager #	When should they be called?	How can they be helpful?

Who might be in the waiting room during the labor and birth?:_____

_____

At what point will you call them?:_____

Would you like any of them to visit you during labor?: ❑ Yes ❑ No

Would you like me to look for ways to include them? If so, what could they do to help? (circle any the couple approves of):

- ◆ call other friends/family regularly during labor

- ◆ get or make a birthday cake

- ◆ get things out of the car

- ◆ set up a little homecoming party at your house

- ◆ bring food in regularly for the coach

- ◆ go to the house, change the sheets, clean up

- ◆ stock the house with groceries

- ◆ run the laundry

- ◆ take pictures of the rest of the family meeting the new baby

Would you like to suggest any other ways to include them?: ❑ Yes ❑ No If so, what?:_____

_____

Who will go to the waiting room to announce the birth?:_____

Do you want people in the waiting room calling your family and friends to announce the birth, or would you like them to wait so that you can do the calling?:_____

Is there anything about any of their personalities or attitudes I should know?:_____

_____

_____

YOUR PREFERENCES DURING LABOR AND BIRTH

The answers to the following questions can help you (the assistant coach) have a better idea of what to expect, and give you ideas of how you can be helpful without disturbing the labor.

What are some things you plan to do to handle pain in labor?:_____

_____

What are her favorite relaxation techniques?:_____

_____

What else will we need to do to help keep her relaxed?:_____

_____

Where does she like to be touched while relaxing?:_____

_____

Where **doesn't** she like to be touched while relaxing?:_____

_____

What words and sounds does she like to hear while relaxing?:_____

_____

What doesn't she want to hear while she's relaxing?:_____

_____

What labor positions does she plan to use?:_____

_____

What birth positions does she plan to try?:_____

_____

_____

*The remaining questions only apply if you are hiring a labor support professional
as your assistant coach.*

MOTHER'S PAST HISTORY (if applicable)

How many other pregnancies have you had?:_____

For each prior pregnancy, list:

Child's Name	Birth Date	Birth Weight	Length of Gestation	Length of Labor and Birth

Have you ever had an unmedicated labor and birth before?: ☐ Yes ☐ No

Were there any complications during any of your previous pregnancies or labors? Please explain:

_____

_____

THIS PREGNANCY

Have you been going for the prenatal appointments regularly?:☐ Yes ☐ No

      Is your health care provider licensed to practice medicine?: ☐ Yes ☐ No

Have you had any complications or warning signs during this pregnancy?: ☐ Yes ☐ No

      Have you discussed all of these with your medical professional?: ☐ Yes ☐ No

Have you been attending childbirth classes regularly?: ☐ Yes ☐ No

Are you doing everything you can to stay healthy and low risk (good nutrition, exercise, education, taking

    responsibility by avoiding harmful things, relaxation)?:_____

SUPPORTING YOUR DESIRE TO HAVE A NATURAL BIRTH

Have you discussed your desire to have an unmedicated birth with your medical team?: ☐ Yes ☐ No

How would you like us (the coach and the assistant coach) to respond if you ask for medication late in labor or

during transition?:_____

_____

There are many things women have found helpful when experiencing pain in labor. They include:

- getting up to walk around
- going to the bathroom
- using relaxation techniques
- having a lot of encouragement
- staying her well hydrated
- trying to find a more efficient or more comfortable position
- taking a shower
- getting a great massage
- applying heat to her lower back and/or abdomen
- taking a spoonful of honey

Would you be willing to try these and/or any other helpful techniques before taking medication? ❏ Yes ❏ No

Some women may ask for medication during labor as a way of getting more help and expressing the intense sensations they are experiencing. When a laboring woman asks her coach or the labor support professional for medication, the typical response is to pour on great coaching techniques and look for natural ways of helping her through it. The way to tell when a woman really needs medication is to see how she behaves in front of her medical team. If a woman asks one of the medical professionals for pain medication, she usually gets it. We cannot contradict your requests.

Remember, unless you _really_ mean it, don't ask the doctor, midwife, or nurse for medication.

ARE WE IN AGREEMENT?

Who referred you to me for professional labor support?:_____

Have you read and discussed this assistant coach's manual?: ❏ Yes ❏ No

Do you understand that your medical professionals are solely responsible for the prediction, diagnosis, and treatment of any complication or risk factor?: ❏ Yes ❏ No

Do you understand that I am not a medical professional and that I do not give medical advice?:❏ Yes ❏ No
  (I can only provide information on natural ways to handle the normal challenges of labor and birth.)

Do you understand that my presence does not guarantee a certain outcome?:❏ Yes ❏ No
  (I can only offer my support and knowledge.)

Do you understand that I will have to leave if asked to by any of your medical professionals?: ☐ Yes ☐ No
(I have no control over their decisions.)

Do you understand that my fee is: $_____

Do you understand the I require a deposit of $_____ by _____ and the balance by _____?

Do you understand that I will make every attempt to be available for your labor and birth but if I become ill or have a family emergency, I will:_____

Do you understand that if your baby comes quickly and you don't call me soon enough or I do not make it there in time, your deposit will be:_____

Do you understand that if you change your minds and decide not to call me to support you during labor and birth, your deposit will be:_____

Do you know that if you have any questions, you can reach me by:_____
_____

The point at which you should call me in labor is:_____

You can reach me in labor by:_____
_____

STAGE	EMOTIONAL SIGNS	BEHAVIOR	PHYSICAL SIGNS
EARLY FIRST STAGE	First emotional signpost:<u>Excitement</u> "Maybe this is it!. . . But then, I'm not sure"	"Putsy-Putsy",stage. Anxiously cleaning, talking, walking, smiling. Walking is important. Many mothers feel restless and need to walk. She may or may not want to move/talk during contractions. She may be hungry.	She may have a bloody show (mucous plug, spotting of blood-tinged mucous or mucous discharge), runny nose, several bowel movements, need to urinate frequently. Note: if heavy bleeding occurs, call birth attendant.
FIRST STAGE	<u>Acceptance</u> "This is it." Confident and committed. "This is a lot of work but I can do it."	Tries various positions and techniques to find what works best and is most comfortable for her. Walking is still important. Looks as if she is working hard but usually prefers to keep busy between contractions.	May be hungry depending on how long the labor has been. May be able to talk and/or move during contractions but it is an effort. She feels many changes occurring in her body, Settling into a pattern.
LATE FIRST STAGE	Second emotional signpost :<u>Seriousness</u> The "do-not-disturb" and "get to work" attitudes.	Losing modesty. May still need to walk, but uses slow deliberate movements. May need to lie down. Appearance of sleep, deeply concentrating. May like sitting on the toilet.	No longer hungry, no longer talkative, even between contractions. She may be sweating, bag of waters may break. She becomes uncomfortable if disturbed, tenses up, or needs to urinate.
TRANSITION	Third emotional signpost: <u>Self-Doubt</u> "This is so hard, I'm so tired. I can't take any more. I give up" <u>Surrender</u>	Confused, unsure, scared, nervous may want to go home, may move around a lot, and give up, may yell at you may be handling things fine.	May be sweaty, shaky, hot then cold, nauseous, may vomit, burp, have cold feet. Bag of waters may break if it hasn't yet.
SECOND STAGE	<u>Calmness</u> and <u>Determination</u> Desire to complete the task. "I want to hold my baby"	No longer modest. Either gradually or suddenly gets the urge to push. Usually more alert and may become more talkative between contractions. May be very tired and might sleep between contractions.	Mucous discharge and some bloody discharge, bag of waters may break if not broken, if it breaks during a contraction, water may burst all over the place. She seems to have gotten a second wind.

These are general guidelines to help you to learn about the normal course of labor. Remember that every labor is different and thsese are only guidelines.

CONTRACTIONS	SENSATIONS	NEEDS	REMINDERS
Generally 10 minutes apart or less. lasting 45-60 seconds and becoming progressively stronger and closer together. Generally do not space out from changing activity.	Strong contractions that peak at about 30 seconds. Possible pressure or cramping feeling. It generally feels better to walk around and keep busy. She may notice many changes in her body at this time.	Keep busy and don't become too excited. This may or may not be actual labor. Have someone with you. Eat if hungry, drink often, get some rest if at all possible.	Walking helps to open the inlet of the pelvis. Adrenaline can slow or stop the labor. If labor stops, don't get discouraged. Rest, eat and go on. This happens often.
Contractions are becoming stronger and more frequent. Generally they are 5 minutes apart or less and lasting around 60 seconds during this stage.	Increasing pressure and fullness in pelvis, backache, cramping feeling across lower back or as with menstrual cramps. May feel stretching in pelvis with sore pubic bone. Pelvis rocks may help.	Support and reassurance. She should not be separated from her coach from now on. Freedom of movement, plenty of space and fresh air are often important. Timing contractions helps.	Conserve your energy, you don't know how long you will be in labor. It is often good to do something fun and entertaining to help pass the time between contractions.
Intense and close, sometimes one on top of another. Generally, (but not always), follow a regular pattern and last 60 seconds or more. May put pressure on bladder causing a need to urinate during contractions.	Hard work, intense, almost overwhelming, you lose track of time, you must concentrate on staying relaxed, tensing up causes pain. Tremendous pressure in pelvis. Feels good to relax completely between contractions and to rest.	Dim lights, comfortable temperature, freedom to move around, peaceful environment, drink and go to the bathroom often. It is important to "give in" and allow the labor to take over.	This is it! You are doing it! Relaxation is the key. Remember the natural alignment plateau. Labor is much more than mere dilation. Be patient, you and your baby need this time.
May become irregular, may double peak, may come one on top of another, may stop completely for a while.	Sensations change greatly, often causing panic, disbelief, and fear. You may feel the baby shifting into alignment with pelvis, a lot of pressure down low. May be the hardest part. It will soon be time to hold your baby.	Reassurance, encouragement, good coaching, various relaxation techniques. Do Not Disturb! Take one contraction at a time. Avoid medication, the hard part is almost over.	Remember: Transition may be the hardest part but it doesn't last long. The baby is coming soon. Your baby is counting on you! Sometimes a spoon full of honey at this point makes the mother feel stronger.
Change to expulsive type. May ease into this stage by pushing only at peaks or can get a sudden urge to push. Usually there is more time between contractions now.	Wait for overwhelming need to bear down. Generally feels better to push and hurts if you don't. Feels sort of like having a huge bowel movement. Most mothers feel a stretching and burning which builds to a tremendous release as the baby is born.	Encouragement and freedom to choose best position. May need a quick lesson on how to push. Everyone should do as mother asks. Give her ice chips or water and reminders to completely relax between contractions.	There are many pushing positions. Squatting and classic are the most efficient. Push to the point of comfort, hold your breath only as long as you are comfortable. This stage can last a few minutes or many hours. *Happy Birth-Day!*

BRADLEY® ENERGY-SAVING TECHNIQUES; THE B.E.S.T. WAY TO HANDLE NORMAL LABORS

The following is a list of energy-saving techniques which thousands of women have found effective and useful during labor. There is no way of predicting how long a labor is going to be, so it is always best to plan on doing everything possible to conserve energy from the very beginning. Even with a fairly short labor, women still use up a tremendous amount of energy. Many obstetricians endorse these suggestions, but each labor is unique, each couple should check with their own birth team. When medical interventions (including Cesareans) become necessary during the course of labors, it is often because the mother became exhausted.

A. Don't pay attention too soon.

Most women experience many series of contractions throughout the weeks and months prior to their actual labors. These natural pregnancy contractions are an important and beneficial part of the body's preparation for birth. It is often a challenge late in pregnancy to determine whether the contractions an expectant mother is experiencing are natural pregnancy contractions (NPC), which mean her body is preparing for labor, or natural labor contractions (NLC), which mean she is in labor.

It is important that the expectant mother not waste her precious energy getting all excited and perhaps even losing sleep over the natural pregnancy contractions. These NPC's are an important part of her body's preparing itself for labor, but are nothing to become alarmed about. Generally, it is best not to be concerned about contractions late in pregnancy until they are ten minutes apart or less, lasting approximately sixty seconds, and are strong enough that the expectant mother can't move or talk during them. These natural labor contractions should gradually become stronger and closer together, and often continue, regardless of change in activity. To get an idea of how strong the contractions are, you can ask her, "Are these contractions strong enough that if you were in the middle of the street and a contraction started, would you have to stop for the contraction?" They will become this strong during the natural course of most labors.

When a situation meets all of the above criteria, then it is probably, but not definitely, labor. Couples who are planning a birth center or hospital birth will probably not want to go in yet. It is generally better to wait until the labor is well-established and the mother is in hard labor before leaving. These are general guidelines which apply to most labors although each situation varies. You should check with your birth team for their suggestions, too.

B. Face your labor calmly.

Whenever an expectant mother thinks she might me in labor, she and her coach should slowly work through this list of five things (provided the labor is not progressing too quickly). 1) Eat something. 2) Have something to drink. 3) Go for a walk. 4) Take a warm bath (provided the bag of waters is still intact). 5) Take a nap. If these are natural pregnancy contractions, they will probably subside by the time they've done all this. If her contractions continue, they should stay calm and attempt to follow her normal daily routine as long as possible. It is important to face the labor calmly because adrenaline, which comes from excitement or fear, can cause even natural labor contractions to become ineffective, more painful, or even stop.

C. Go back home if you arrive at your birth place too early.

Most first-time parents end up going to their birth place once or twice before their real labor starts. As Dr. Bradley explains, "It's not that you are crazy or that you're not quite bright; your medical team probably won't know if you're in labor either. They will observe you for a while to see if the labor continues and if you progress." Couples should try not to be too anxious or concerned. If they are not sure whether or not they're in labor, they should call their Bradley® teacher or their health care provider and discuss it. The only way to know for sure they are having natural pregnancy contractions or natural labor contractions is to wait and see if the labor continues to progress and the baby is born.

Regardless of which type of contractions they are having, good coaching and lots of support are important. When they think it's time, couples sometimes meet their health care provider at the office first, before checking in at the hospital or birth center. This can help avoid the problem of arriving at the birth place too early. Couples who go straight to the hospital or birth center sometimes ask to delay all of the admitting procedures (blood and urine tests, paperwork, putting on a gown, etc.) until they have gotten settled and everyone agrees it is far enough into the labor for her to stay. Mother's who have already gone through all these procedures are emotionally committed and often want to stay, even if the medical staff is encouraging them to go home.

Dr. Victor Berman, a well-known obstetrician who specializes in natural childbirth, encourages women to follow what is known as "Berman's Law," which says that most women should not stay in the hospital or birth center if they are less than five centimeters dilated. This is a very good guideline, most of the time. Women who are less than five centimeters and still showing early labor signs (both physical and behavioral), probably are too early, especially since most hospitals impose time limits for labor and birth. Once in a rare while, a woman is three or four centimeters, but very close to being ready to push. Her physical and behavioral signs show it, and they are more reliable than cervical dilation. When a woman's physical and behavioral signs indicate that she is in late first stage, she should consider staying at her birthplace regardless of what her cervix shows.

D. Use relaxation to handle contractions.

Tensing up during contractions wastes valuable energy and can cause a tremendous amount of totally unnecessary pain. It is much better to use deep relaxation techniques, which are more effective and less painful. Relaxation should be practiced regularly during pregnancy. With the proper training and plenty of practice, women will be able to relax automatically and completely as contractions begin, and in response to their coach's voice and touch.

Relaxation is the key to the Bradley Method® and can be very helpful even for women who have not practiced much, prior to labor. But, it is the couple who has faithfully practiced the relaxation techniques taught in class that can realize fully the incredible benefits of deep relaxation in labor.

E. Use normal abdominal breathing during labor.

Each expectant mother already knows how to breathe. They have been doing a good job of it all for a long time. They do not need to be taught how to breathe. Breathing automatically becomes more rapid when a lot of energy is exerted. It automatically slows when the body is calm and relaxed. People do not have to worry about adjusting their breathing through the many situations they face in life, and there is no reason for expectant mothers to worry about it either. Their breathing will automatically adjust itself in labor, too.

The Bradley Method® does not teach chest-breathing and altered breathing patterns because they use up a tremendous amount of energy, and are more likely to cause hyperventilation, which has been shown to be dangerous for both the mother and the baby. "Breathing" is not as effective as relaxation is in dealing with contractions. So laboring moms should, relax and let their breathing take care of itself!

F. Walk during labor.

Dr. Roberto Caldeyro-Barcia has studied walking during labor and found that it shortens labor by an average of twenty-eight percent. Walking opens the inlet of the pelvis, so the baby has more room to get down into and maneuver through the pelvis. Women also seem to have more energy and experience less pain when they are up and around than when they've been lying down for a long time. Laboring mothers who get up and walk around are usually glad they did!

G. Keep drinking during labor.

Most medical professionals we've worked with encourage women to keep drinking during labor because drinking a large glass of water or juice every hour helps to replace fluids, prevent dehydration and keep the body functioning properly. While in labor, women work very hard. It may be some of the hardest work they ever do in their lives. Giving birth is an athletic event. The body depends on fluids to keep it functioning properly. A lot of fluids are lost through perspiration and discharge. It is important to keep drinking during labor.

H. Eat if you're hungry.

Dehydration during labor can cause a woman's blood pressure to go up, her temperature to rise, and her pulse rate to increase—all clearly undesirable conditions in labor.

Eating is a very important way people store energy and keep up their strength. Laboring women use up a tremendous amount of energy in labor. They should be encouraged to tune-in to their body. The laboring woman should ask herself, "Am I hungry?" and, "What am I hungry for?" Eating will often cause natural pregnancy contractions to subside and may help to help prevent premature labor.

Many women are quite hungry in early labor. They eat a good meal and have the strength to labor for hours, then go on to give birth to their babies. Once in hard labor, most women are no longer hungry, in which case they probably should not eat.

Some hospitals still restrict food intake of mothers in labor. If a mother needs some extra energy in hard labor, some juice, hard candy, or a spoonful of honey will generally do the trick.

I. Sleep if you're sleepy.

No one knows how long their labor is going to take. Laboring women should be encouraged to sleep any time they can sleep. They will need the energy later! It is possible for most women to sleep between contractions. If a woman is having regular contractions, her coach should wake her thirty seconds or so before the next contraction starts. This gives her some warning that the contraction is coming and prevents her from having to deal with the huge challenge of waking up at the peak of a contraction.

Women should not be afraid to sleep during labor. Good strong contractions will wake them. Unmedicated women do not sleep through having babies. Some labors progress slowly because the mother is tired and needs some sleep.

We know many mothers who went through long first stages but, during transition, their contractions stopped completely. These mothers took this opportunity to get some rest. Most of them slept for about two hours. When they awoke, they felt refreshed and went immediately into second stage and pushed their babies out.

Women who are very tired in second stage can sleep between contractions then, too. They are glad to get even a few minutes rest.

J. Stay active as long as you can.

Just because she is in labor, is no reason a woman should lie down and act sick. Just because she has been assigned a hospital bed is no reason for her to feel she has to be in it all of the time.

The side relaxation position should only be used if the contractions have become so strong that the laboring mother must lie down and concentrate on relaxation or if she is tired and needs to sleep.

Keeping occupied with games, books, music, or whatever the laboring woman enjoys, will be helpful during the early part of the labor. Going for a walk outside and taking a bath or shower are often invigorating for them. Lying down for long periods of time can cause mothers to become bored and tired, and that's not a good thing in labor.

Sure, labor is a lot of very hard work, but it can be fun too! Couples should try to enjoy this precious time as they labor and give birth to their babies.

K. Try taking a warm bath or shower.

When going through hard labor, perhaps just before leaving for the birth place, the laboring mother might want to try getting in warm water. This is a good idea provided the bag of waters is still intact and the temperature does not exceed body temperature. It often reduces pain, encourages deep relaxation, and speeds labor. Being submerged in warm water seems to help women "let go". This is an important part of giving birth. So for labor, when the going gets tough, the tough take a bath!

Some women enjoy going into a spa or hot tub during labor. Some hospitals and birth centers have installed special labor tubs that women can use. Before going into any spa or hot tub any time during pregnancy, the mother should be sure that it is clean, well-maintained, and that the temperature is kept below body temperature.

L. Avoid taking medication.

The drugs and medications used in childbirth today are neither as safe nor as effective as most people believe. They pose a definite danger to the mother and the baby, and are not necessary for the vast majority of couples who take Bradley® classes.

Taking medication during labor can be a waste of time and energy. One of the most common drugs used in labor is Demerol. Although often referred to as "just a little relaxer," it is not as harmless as it sounds. Demerol is a narcotic, the same family as heroin. Besides its many effects on the mother and baby, Demerol relaxes the uterus. Think about it for a minute. Is this what needs to be done in labor? The uterus is a large bag of muscles which contracts to open the cervix and expel the baby. Relaxing the uterus is likely to slow the progress of labor. Often, the medication leaves a mother groggy and unable to handle her contractions well; therefore, she experiences more pain. Sometimes mothers who take medication must wait until it wears off before they can continue progressing.

Taking medication in labor involves some risk, and is best left for the case of a complication where the benefits outweigh the risks.

Dr. Bradley says, "the loving encouragement from a trained labor coach can do more for the comfort and relaxation of his wife than any amount of medication." So keep up the good coaching, and avoid the medication.

M. Continued enthusiastic encouragement is essential.

Becoming depressed or discouraged is one of the worst things that can happen to a laboring couple! The work they are doing is extremely important. Yes, it's difficult and, perhaps quite painful, but it is important! Their baby needs this labor and the mother is the only one who can give it to him or her. She needs this labor too. Everyone supporting her should be encouraging so she won't sell herself short. "You can do it! Just hang on."

The laboring woman can get the most out of every contraction by completely relaxing and letting go. She should not become discouraged even if the dilation is slow or seems to have stalled. Her coach should remind her about the natural alignment plateau; a naturally occurring phenomenon that they learned about in their Bradley® classes. Progress is being made with each passing contraction. There is much more to labor than mere dilation.

Couples must not get hung-up on time. Some labors move quickly, others take a long time. Women who have long labors need to stay positive. Instead of thinking of the labor as having gone on for days. They should focus only on the length of time they have been in late first stage labor. Even if a woman has been in early first stage labor on and off for two days, as long as she has been careful to conserve her energy, it has been two days with lots of rest and plenty of support and attention from her coach, mixed with occasional contractions. She should be ready and able to face the hard work in front of her when it comes. She should count only the length of time she spends in late first stage labor. Only the strong, all-encompassing contractions when she shows definite active labor behavioral signs are the ones that she should count when she considers how long she has been in labor.

People who support women in labor need to consider, "Is the mother all right, physically? Are the baby's vital signs good?" As long as there are no clear indications of a complication and women are careful to conserve their energy, they can continue to follow the natural course of labor.

Allowing a labor to follow its natural course may not be easy, but it does make a difference! This is the way that most women can do the best thing for themselves and their babies. They would not be as well off with some medication or by having a Cesarean section for no medical reason. Each laboring woman has only one chance to give birth to that baby. They will not be in labor forever. They will give birth and then be able to rest. They need to be reminded, "allowing your labor to follow it's natural course is so important. You're doing a great job! You're a great mommy!"

There are good reasons for everything in nature, and there are good reasons for long labors when they happen. Every minute is worthwhile. Every contraction is beneficial. Throughout each labor, the mother is doing some of the most important work that can ever be done. She deserves all the credit and praise in the world.

N. Be aware of natural, effective techniques to speed labor.

Sometimes labors go on and on, which is probably beneficial in some way as long as people are patient and the mother is careful to conserve her energy. If it becomes necessary to speed the labor for some reason, there are a few very effective techniques a coach can try.

1) Encourage the mother to get up and walk. Walking opens the inlet of the pelvis to get the baby down and is an effective means of speeding labor. 2) Ask the mother to try using nipple stimulation. She can just use her fingers or the heel of her hand and rub up and down over one or both of her nipples. Right through her gown is fine. Nipple stimulation

has been shown to be an effective way to accelerate labor, and has been used for centuries. Nipple stimulation usually results in more powerful, more frequent contractions almost immediately. Continue using stimulation between each contraction, as long as is necessary. 3) Another means of accelerating labor is to use pressure. The mother can push her thumb up against her palate (the roof of her mouth), an action similar to sucking your thumb. This is a pressure point that seems to stimulate labor. 4) Do what is necessary to reduce the mother's fear and anxieties. Sometimes, all that she needs is to discuss her fears and be assured that she is not alone. Some mothers who go to the hospital too soon and find that they can't relax well there may need to go home for a while, so that they can "give in" and let labor take over. Other mothers find that they are so uneasy at home that they cannot relax well and "give in" to their labors until they are in the hospital. Each situation must be evaluated individually.

So, if it becomes necessary to speed labor, the coach should first talk with the mother. Find out if any changes are necessary so that she can fully relax, "give in" to her labor, let her body open up and give birth to her baby. Then, recharge the mother in some way (a spoonful of honey, a cool drink, a warm shower, for example). Instill in her a positive, enthusiastic attitude. Remind her, "It is time to get down to work and have this baby." Next, go for a walk outside, around the corridors—someplace as spacious and private as possible. Most mothers do not like feeling confined, and feel strange rubbing their nipples and sucking their thumb in public.

As she walks and does some nipple stimulation and then sucks her thumb briefly, she will most likely have a contraction. When the contraction begins, she should lean forward against her coach and let him support her. She should just hang loose and limp, completely relaxed, and concentrate on letting go and opening up. Each contraction should be followed by enthusiastic encouragement. "We're really getting somewhere. You are doing a great job! Let's do it again!"

Again, she would begin walking at a good pace, stimulate her nipples, and suck her thumb. Again, it is likely to result in a good, strong, effective contraction. The mother will probably be having contractions that are much more powerful by this time. She may comment that these contractions are more painful, and that's a positive sign. The stronger the contractions are, the sooner the baby will be born.

These very effective techniques are likely to bring results. Although it is sometimes necessary to continue this way for many hours, changes may also come about very quickly. Coaches should watch for the pain which moves lower and lower down her back or in front against her pubic bone and the feeling of tremendous pressure low in her pelvis. These are all great signs. They mean that the baby is coming down. Coaches must keep up with an enthusiastic attitude and continue with these techniques as long as necessary. It is important to remind the laboring woman to drink and go to the bathroom often. Take one contraction at a time and watch for progress.

O. Push only when you're ready to push.

Laboring women should try not to push until they feel an undeniable urge to push. Many women waste energy pushing before they are ready. Sometimes a mother is encouraged to push too soon (before her urge to push comes). This can be a problem, because the baby can be pushed down in a bad position, making a normal delivery difficult or even impossible. When a woman is in hard labor, relaxing and handling her contractions well, she and her baby may need some more time before pushing, even if she is completely dilated.

Once in a while a woman does not recognize her urge to push. She grunts and groans, tenses up, can no longer relax well, and has a lot of very painful contractions. In this case, the coach might need to encourage her to try pushing gently and see how it feels.

When done correctly, pushing can be an effective means of pain control. When a mother begins actively pushing, she should be sure that it feels better to push than not to push. On occasion, a woman will give birth without pushing at all. These are all normal variations.

P. Use positive pushing techniques.

There are a few important points coaches need to remind the laboring mother of when she starts pushing. 1) Push to the point of comfort. She should exert only the amount of energy necessary at the time. This is not a contest. She should push at her own speed. There are a lot of very important and beneficial processes going on inside of her body during second stage. It is all right if she takes her time. 2) Hold your breath only as long as is comfortable. She will need to take several breaths during a contraction. Her body will let her know how often to breathe. If she pays attention, she'll do just fine. 3)While you're pushing, relax everything except the muscles necessary to push and hold yourself in the pushing position you've chosen. She should not: tense her face, clench her jaw, tense her hands or feet, or tense across her buttocks. The coach should tell her to "let go" with each push. "Push down and out. Let your body open up. Let your baby come down and out." The perineum should bulge during pushes. 4) Between contractions, let go of your legs, drop your arms, lean back and completely relax. She is likely to have longer rest periods between contractions now. She should take advantage of this time and recoup her energy. Some women even doze between contractions and that's fine.

Q. Be aware of effective pushing positions.

Mothers should be free to use whatever pushing positions they prefer. If the mother is running out of energy or a time limit is imposed on her, she might need to use one of the most effective pushing positions to speed her second stage.

Squatting opens the outlet of the pelvis by at least ten to fifteen percent. A modified squat on a labor bed or a delivery table is not quite as effective, but still may be useful. Using a full squatting position, coupled with breath-holding and positive pushing techniques, is probably the fastest way to push a baby out.

We believe that it is best to allow each labor to follow its natural course, if at all possible. Once in a while these aggressive pushing techniques become important; so all couples should be aware of them.

Have a Very Happy Birth-Day!

To learn more about the Bradley Method® natural childbirth, contact your local Bradley® instructor. Have a very happy birth-day!

ARE YOU READY TO DO YOUR B.E.S.T?

Can you complete this questionnaire? The answers are from the preceding section.

A. DON'T PAY ATTENTION TOO SOON

1. What signs can help a woman decide whether she is in labor or just having natural pregnancy contractions?

2. At what point should her coach begin timing contractions?:

3. What signs should he be looking for to help him decide when it is time to take her to the birth place?

Contractions:

Behavioral Signs:

Physical Signs:

B. FACE YOUR LABOR CALMLY

1. When an expectant mother thinks she might be in labor, what five things should she do?:

2. What can adrenaline (which can come from excitement, fear, anxiety, etc.) do to a labor?:

C. GO BACK HOME IF YOU ARRIVE AT YOUR BIRTH PLACE TOO EARLY

1. Whom should the expectant mother or her coach call to discuss their situation when they think they might be in labor?:

2. What does "Berman's Law" say?:

D. USE RELAXATION TO HANDLE CONTRACTIONS

1. Tensing up during contractions will waste _____ and cause _____ pain.

2. What is the key to The Bradley Method®?

3. Couples should _____ every day so that the expectant mother becomes so good at relaxing that she can relax immediately and completely in response to her coach's _____ and _____.

E. USE NORMAL, ABDOMINAL BREATHING

1. What are three reasons The Bradley Method® doesn't teach altered breathing patterns?

2. ❑ True or ❑ False: If you relax and tune-in to your body, your breathing will take care of itself.

F. WALK DURING LABOR

1. Dr. Roberto Caldeyro-Barcia has determined that walking can _____ labors by an average of 28%.

2. Walking helps to open the _____ of the pelvis to help the baby come down.

G. KEEP DRINKING DURING LABOR

1. What does drinking one large glass of liquid every hour during labor help to do?:

2. Why is it important to avoid dehydration during labor?:

H. EAT IF YOU'RE HUNGRY

1. Eating during early labor can help you to store _____ and keep your _____ up.

2. What two questions can a woman ask herself when trying to decide if she should eat during labor?:

3. If the laboring mother's intake has been restricted but she needs to raise her blood sugar, what can she try?:

I. SLEEP IF YOU'RE SLEEPY

1. If you can sleep, then _____.

2. What can a coach do for a woman who's sleeping between contractions so that the next contraction does not take her by surprise?:

3. Do women ever take a break and sleep for an hour or two during the course of a normal labor?:

4. Do women ever sleep between contractions in second (pushing) stage?:

J. STAY ACTIVE AS LONG AS YOU CAN

1. Should a woman in early labor lie down and try not to move? What effect could this have on the labor?:

2. When should a laboring woman begin to use the side relaxation position?

3. What could the mother and her coach do during early labor to pass the time and stay active?:

K. TRY TAKING A WARM BATH OR SHOWER
1. When would it be especially helpful to labor in warm water?:

2. In what case should a mother check with her birth attendant before taking a bath or going into a spa or hot tub?:

3. When in a spa or hot tub, it is best to keep the temperature below _____ _____.

4. What does getting into warm water generally do for a woman in labor?:

L. AVOID TAKING MEDICATION
1. Are there any potentially dangerous side effects to the mother and baby from the drugs which can be used during childbirth?:

2. Do most mothers trained in The Bradley Method® need to take medication during labor and/or birth?:

3. Medication, as well as the various life-saving techniques which can be used in labor, are best left for the case of a true complication where the _____ outweigh the _____.

4. According to Dr. Bradley, the loving encouragement from a trained coach can do more for the _____ and _____ of his wife than any amount of _____.

M. CONTINUED ENTHUSIASTIC ENCOURAGEMENT IS ESSENTIAL
1. What can laboring couples do to help prevent themselves from becoming depressed and discouraged during a long labor?:

2. What must the mother do in order to get the most out of every contraction?:

3. As long as there are no indications of a complication and the mother is careful to _____ her _____, she can continue to follow the natural course of her labor.

N. BE AWARE OF NATURAL, EFFECTIVE TECHNIQUES TO SPEED LABOR

1. List four things that are likely to speed up a labor.:

2. What discomforts for the mother are also signs that the baby is coming down?:

O. PUSH ONLY WHEN YOU'RE READY TO PUSH

1. Why is it important for the mother to wait for her urge to push?:

2. What guideline can help you to determine if it's time to push?:

P. USE POSITIVE PUSHING TECHNIQUES

1. During second stage, the mother should push to the point of _____ and hold her breath only as long as is _____.

2. What should the mother do between contractions during second stage?:

Q. BE AWARE OF THE MOST EFFECTIVE PUSHING POSITIONS

1. What position can the mother use to open the outlet of the pelvis by at least 10-15%?:

2. What other position can also help to open the outlet of the pelvis but is generally more acceptable in a hospital environment?:

HAVE A VERY HAPPY BIRTH-DAY!

Remember these are suggestions for normal labors. Thousands of women have used these techniques and found them effective and useful during labor. Many obstetricians endorse these suggestions, but each labor is unique. Each couple must check with their health care provider to discuss their particular case.

UNDERSTANDING TRANSITION

The following is written to the coach. Its purpose is to help coaches understand and better prepare for the emotional challenge that sometimes comes during the transition stage. As an assistant coach, you may also benefit from a greater understanding of what a mother experiences during a challenging transition.

♦ She may feel out of control, but that's understandable; the woman does not control the labor.

♦ She may feel tired, but that's understandable; she's been working very had and she will soon get a burst of new energy.

♦ She may feel confused, upset, and unsure, but that's understandable; transition is the time of confusion, it will soon pass.

♦ She may not know what to do anymore, but that's understandable; and that's why she has you.

♦ She may say it really hurts, but that's understandable; she's having a baby! Soon the baby will be born and it will all have been worth it.

♦ She may cry, but that's understandable; she's going through a very emotional time, but she has your shoulder to cry on and your strength to see her through.

♦ She may say she needs "something for the pain," but that's understandable; transition is the most common time for women to ask for medication. You know how to help her through without the drugs; you are the "something" that she needs.

♦ She may criticize you, but that's understandable; she's in transition and she knows that you will not be offended.

♦ She may think that she's not doing a very good job, but that's understandable; she's going through a time of self-doubt. Labor is such a big challenge, it is never exactly what you expected. She needs you to remind her of what a good job she's doing.

♦ She may say that she really wants the drugs, but that's understandable; transition can be difficult, but it does not last long. By the time the medication could take effect, transition would probably be over and she won't want to miss the wonderful sensations and feelings of accomplishment that come from giving birth without drugs.

RELAXING WORDS AND PHRASES

Good verbal coaching is something many mothers rely on during labor. You may be asked to take over briefly for the coach when he needs to eat or use the bathroom. During the short time he is out of the room, she may be a little more uncomfortable and need a lot of verbal support. The following is a list of relaxing words and phrases that many women have found helpful during labor. If at some point during labor the coach becomes tired and can no longer think of what to say, refer to this list and give him some good suggestions.

Relaxing Words:	Describe Contractions As:
relax	strong
let go	powerful
give in	effective
sink	efficient
slip	good
slide	positive
flow	an opportunity to make progress
float	bringing us closer to the birth
melt	
down	**Praise**
out	Good job!
through	Great work!
loose	Excellent!
limp	I'm so proud of you!
open	I believe in you!
release	You handled that wonderfully!
drift	That's the way!
glide	You're relaxing beautifully!
slow	Super job!
easy	You're such a good mommy!

CONTRACTION SCRIPTS

Coaches get extensive training and lots of practice in their Bradley® class. They learn how to help the mother handle her contractions and what to say to provide good verbal support for her. The following contraction scripts have been included in this manual to help you get a better understanding of the kind of things a coach will say during contractions, and to better prepare you for any times you would be asked to take over briefly for the coach. The relaxing words and phrases on page 85 is similar, but these scripts spell out, word for word, everything you would say during a sixty second contraction. This can also be a helpful resource if the coach becomes tired and needs suggestions of what to say.

How to use contraction scripts:

When the script says, ':00' it indicates the beginning of the contraction; the point at which you begin timing. During this time, the uterus pulls forward and begins contracting (tightening).

When it says, ':15', it indicates that the contraction has gone on for fifteen seconds. The contraction is building in intensity now; contracting (squeezing) harder and harder. At this point, you say, "fifteen seconds" and the words that follow it.

When it says, ':30', it indicates that the contraction has gone on for thirty seconds. This is the peak (the strongest part) of the contraction. This is the most challenging time. At this point, you say, "thirty seconds" and the words that follow it.

When it says, ':45', it indicates that the contraction has gone on for forty-five seconds. By now, most contractions will begin to subside. At this point, you say, "forty-five seconds" and the words that follow it.

When it says, ':60', it indicates that the contraction has gone on for sixty seconds. Most contractions end at this point. Wait for her to indicate that it is over. Continue coaching and encouraging her until then. Notice that every contraction ends with some praise for the mother.

All of these words must be said with a calm, relaxing voice. The tone of your voice, the pace of your speech, the touch of your hands, everything must convey relaxation.

:00	*Concentrate on relaxation as you ease into this contraction.*
:15	*The stronger the contraction, the more you need to relax.*
:30	*This is the peak of this contraction. You are relaxing well and making a lot of progress right now.*
:45	*This contraction should gradually subside now.*
:60	*Good work!*

:00	*Welcome this contraction by relaxing completely. That's the way.*
:15	*Let it go. Feel all the tension melt away. You're doing a great job!*
:30	*This is the peak of the contraction. The more you relax now, the more progress you'll make and the more progress you make with this contraction, the fewer you'll have to have.*
:45	*Relax deeper and deeper as the contraction begins to subside. Excellent!*
:60	*Great job!*

:00	*As the contraction begins, feel any tension in your body melt away.*
:15	*Think about your body becoming comfortably heavy as you sink deeper and deeper into a relaxed state.*
:30	*As the contraction peaks, release, let go and give in to it. Let this powerful contraction do it's important work.*
:45	*You are doing very well. Everything is fine.*
:60	*I'm so proud of you!*

:00	*Here we go. Relax into the contraction. Open up, and breathe slowly. Let all the tension flow out of your body and float with this contraction.*
:15	*Use slow and easy, abdominal breathing. Breathe in and out slowly. Think of yourself as a leaf, floating on a stream.*
:30	*You've reached the peak of this contraction. Concentrate on your hands being loose and limp and relaxed.*
:45	*As the contraction subsides, feel your body sink deeper and deeper into the bed.*
:60	*Excellent!*

:00	*Welcome the contraction. Relax and let go. Good job.*
:15	*The stronger the contraction is, the more you relax. Very good. Think about your hands being loose, and limp, and relaxed.*
:30	*This is the strongest and most beneficial part of this contraction. You are making good progress right now. Completely relax so you can get the most out of this contraction.*
:45	*As the contraction begins to subside, concentrate on opening wide the way for the baby. Allow the baby to sink deeper and deeper into your pelvis.*
:60	*Wonderful job!*

:00	*I am here with you and I will help you. Now, start by relaxing your head, your eyes, nose, mouth, jaw and all the way down your neck.*
:15	*Very good. Relax across your shoulders and down to your elbows. Think all the tension down from your elbows, through to your wrists, and out of your fingertips.*
:30	*This is the most effective part of this contraction. You're doing a great job. Relax your upper back and your chest. Relax your lower back and relax extremely under your abdomen; let go of the baby.*
:45	*Relax across your hips and down your legs to your knees. Relax through to your ankles and down and out your toes.*
:60	*You're doing such a good job!*

:00	As this contraction begins, relax your whole body. Let your uterus do what it needs to do. Let it go.
:15	As the contraction gets stronger and stronger, you relax deeper and deeper.
:30	Relax your Kegel muscle and all the way through your birth canal so the baby can slide lower and lower as he/she gradually makes his/her way out.
:45	The baby is fine. You are fine. Everything is fine. You just focus on the important work that you are doing. We will take care of everything else.
:60	You do this so well!

:00	Begin by relaxing and letting go. Concentrate on feeling you body sink deeper and deeper as you relax. Concentrate on your hands being loose and limp, comfortably relaxed.
:15	Use slow and easy abdominal breathing. Breathe in and out slowly. Relax all around your uterus, relax behind it, and under it.
:30	Relax and open the pathway for your baby. As you feel the stretch, encourage the pressure. The baby will work his/her way down and out through there. This is very challenging. You're doing great.
:45	You're almost done. Just a few more seconds to go. Feel your body relax deeper and deeper as the contraction subsides.
:60	You are doing such a great job! You're such a good mommy!

WHY HAVE A NATURAL BIRTH?

The following article is from Doris Haire, president of the American Foundation for Maternal and Child Health. She is also a past chairwoman of the National Women's Health Network.

Caution needed with labor drugs

Many people mistakenly believe that childbirth medications are "perfectly safe".

Until fairly recently, the administration of drugs to a woman during labor to relieve her discomfort or pain or to stimulate her contractions was thought to have little or no lasting effect on the mother or her baby. Limited technology allowed many obstetricians to assume that the placenta was a reasonably effective barrier between the mother's circulation and that of the unborn infant. Some wishful thinking obstetricians even told their maternity patients that anesthesia would protect the fetal brain from birth trauma!

All medications given during labor reach the baby's blood and brain within minutes or seconds.

One only has to read the manufacturer's information leaflet of any of the drugs commonly given to women during labor to realize that all of these drugs enter the blood and brain of the baby within seconds or minutes and place the mother and her baby at significant risk. How often do drug adverse effects occur? No one really knows, for the FDA does not require a doctor to report an adverse drug reaction, even if the patient dies.

Unborn babies are particularly vulnerable.

During the hours that surround an infant's birth the brain is particularly vulnerable to drug-induced trauma and permanent injury. Other major organ systems are essentially formed by the first three or four months of pregnancy. It is the nerve circuitry of the brain and central nervous system of the fetus that is rapidly developing as labor begins, making these awesomely complex structures vulnerable to permanent damage from drugs and procedures administered to the mother during that time.

While the fetus is connected to the mother's circulatory system, she helps to eliminate the drugs from both systems. However, if a drug is frequently or continuously administered to the mother during labor, there is a tendency for the drug to accumulate in the maternal and fetal blood and brain.

Once the infant is born and the cord is clamped, the newborn's immature metabolic and endocrine systems cannot readily break down and excrete the drugs. Therefore, the trapped drugs, or their potent metabolies, may continue to circulate in the newborn's blood and brain for several days or longer.

The effects on an infant can last weeks or longer.

Is there any lasting effect of these drugs on the neurologic development of the exposed infant? A six-week follow-up evaluation by Deborah Rosenblatt in the United Kingdom of infants exposed to bupivacaine epidurals during labor demonstrated significant and consistent effects of the drug throughout the six-week assessment period. The initial effects were cyanosis (decreased oxygenation of the infant) and unresponsiveness. The infant's visual skills, alertness, motor organization, ability to control states of consciousness and physiological response to stress were adversely affected. A more recent four-week follow-up investigation carried out by Carol Sepkoski, T. Berry Brazelton and their colleagues at Harvard University resulted in similar findings.

Having an epidural during labor drastically increases the likelihood that a cesarean will become necessary.

We have long known that epidural anethesia increases the likelihood that the baby will ahve to be extracted by forceps or vacuum extractor, with all the hazards those procedures imply. Now James Thorp and his colleagues at the University of Missouri have shown that the rate of Cesarean sections is increased tenfold when a woman is given an epidural block during labor. If the baby has been exposed to pain-relieving medication administered to the mother over several hours and then receives additional stronger drugs necessary for a cesarean, the baby is even more likely to have breathing problems.

Narcotics are commonly given during labor.

While narcotics and narcotic-like drugs such as meperidine, butorphonal, nalbuphine or other potent pain-relieving drugs have less adverse effects on the progress of labor, they too can depress the neurologic function of the newborn and increase the likelihood that the baby will need to be resuscitated.

Using The Bradley Method®, over 80% of mothers have unmedicated births.

What can you do to protect your baby from the harmful effects of obstetric drugs? First, tell your doctor you want to read the package inserts of the drugs he or she might want to use in your case. If the indications section of the package insert does not mention relevant words, such as "pregnancy, labor, delivery," then the FDA has NOT approved the drug for such use.

Every life has only one beginning. You owe it to yourself and your baby to make it the very best possible start.

The above article is included in this manual with the permission of Doris B. Haire. Visit her website at www.aimsusa.org.

LOOKING FOR WAYS TO SUPPORT THE LABORING COUPLE

Whenever you (the assistant coach) are unsure of what you should be doing, step back and open your eyes. Start in one corner and glance around the room. You won't make it all the way around before you find something that needs to be done. Ask yourself:

♦ Is the lighting too bright?
♦ Is the temperature comfortable for the mother?
♦ Should you get him a wash cloth to put on her face?
♦ Does anything need to be cleaned up?
♦ Is her sipper bottle filled?
♦ Has she been drinking enough?
♦ Would she like a hot water bottle for her abdomen or lower back?
♦ Are you keeping adequate notes of contractions and other things?
♦ Has she been going to the bathroom frequently enough?
♦ What is the coach drinking?
♦ Does he need some food now?"

Be observant, find a need and then fill it. While you're doing one thing, look around and ask yourself, "what's next?"

The following situations give very specific examples of ways an assistant coach can find a lot of things that need to be done. While you are supporting the laboring couple, you will need to apply whatever ideas are appropriate at that time. Keep your eyes open, you will find that there is plenty to do.

Situation #1: The mother is in late first stage labor. She is up walking around between contractions. When each contraction begins, she stops. The coach reminds her to put her feet wide apart so that she feels more stable, and to bend her knees slightly to relieve pressure from her lower back. He gently moves so that he is standing in front of her, then cuddles her into his chest and, once she is stable and he is ready, says, "let it go" in a deeply relaxing tone. She responds by relaxing into his arms and letting him support her. When the contraction is over, he asks if she needs a boost. If she does, he slowly counts to three, then boosts her up without letting go of her. He holds on to her as she gets her balance. Next, he gives her two things; praise, and a sip of water (or juice, or whatever she is drinking). When the mother is ready, she begins walking again and the coach follows her lead, walking beside her at whatever pace she sets, supporting and encouraging her as she moves.

Suggestions of ways the assistant coach might support this couple:
♦ Walk behind them carrying the sipper bottle.
♦ Offer to stroke her hair during the contraction.
♦ Offer to rub her back during the contraction (the coach probably cannot reach it).
♦ Offer to use long flowing stokes down her arms during the contraction.
♦ Encourage and support them.

- Time the contractions. Tell the coach when it's been 15 seconds, 30 seconds, 45 seconds, and sixty seconds. (He probably can't see his watch in this position.)
- Stand behind the mom when the contraction is over, so when he boosts her up you can hold her shoulders and help stabilize her.
- Keep the sipper bottle filled. (Once it gets lower than 1/3 full, it can be hard for her to get anything out of it.)
- Tell her, "Excellent work!"
- Tell him, "You're good at this!"

Situation #2: *The mother is in late first stage. Her bag of waters has already broken or is leaking and she is up walking between contractions. As each contraction begins, she stops in front of a counter-top, dresser, or something she can lean over on to. The coach lays a chux pad or towel on the floor in front of her and asks her to step forward onto it. He reminds her to keep a wide stance so she feels more stable. He supports her as she leans over and adjusts her position. At 10 seconds into the contraction, or whenever the mother is stable and ready, the coach says, "let it go" in a deeply relaxing tone. She responds by releasing and allowing her weight to be supported by whatever she is leaning on. During the contraction, the coach encourages her to open up and relax extremely under her abdomen and through her birth canal. He encourages her to welcome the oozing, slippery, sliding feeling and relax so completely that water spills forward during the contraction. When the contraction is over, he asks if she needs a boost. If she does, he slowly counts to three, then boosts her up to a standing position. He holds on to her as she becomes stable. Next he gives her some praise, and a sip of water (or juice, or whatever she is drinking). Then he takes a tissue and wipes off any fluid that has run down her leg(s), and supports her as she starts walking again.*

Suggestions of ways the assistant coach might support this couple:
- Keep an eye on the clock. Let the coach know approximately 30 seconds before the next contraction is likely to begin so they can position themselves near the object she is leaning over on.
- Carry the chux pad or towel and the box of tissues for him.
- Lay the chux pad or towel down where they need it.
- Lay a pillow down on top of the object she is leaning on (to make it softer and more comfortable).
- Stroke down her arms during contractions.
- Encourage both of them.
- Reassure her that this is just part of being in labor and no reason to be embarrassed.
- Carry the sipper bottle for him.
- Wipe off her leg(s) after the contraction so the coach can hold on to her and stay up by her face.
- Remind her that when water spills forward it usually indicates progress (the baby is moving down).
- Tell her, "You're doing a great job!"
- Tell him, "Good work, coach!"

Situation #3: It is late first stage. The mother is in the shower. The coach is standing outside the shower encouraging and coaching her. When each contraction begins, he reminds her to put her feet wide apart so that she feels more stable, and to bend her knees slightly to relieve pressure from her lower back. She leans against the wall of the shower. He rubs her back and coaches her through the contraction. He asks her to concentrate on relaxing her muscles as she feels the water streaming down her body. he stands ready to help her if she relaxes so much that she begins to slide down the wall. When the contraction is over, he asks if she needs a boost. If she does, he slowly counts to three and gently boosts her up to a standing position and holds on to her as she becomes stable. He follows each contraction by giving her some praise and a sip of water (or juice, or whatever she is drinking).

Suggestions of ways the assistant coach might support this couple:
- Get a towel for the coach to dry off with.
- Be sure a dry towel and a clean gown is ready whenever the mother decides to get out.
- Get him a change of clothes if he needs it (perhaps he would rather wear his bathing suit).
- Keep her sipper bottle filled.
- Answer the phone if it rings.
- Take care of anything that needs to be done outside of that room. (Do they have plenty of whatever she likes to drink? Does the coach need something to eat or drink? Does anything need to be cleaned up? Is the bed ready for when she decides to lay down? Would this be a good time for you to sit or lie down and get some rest?)
- Tell her, "You're doing great! Hang in there, you can do it!"
- Tell him, "She's lucky to have you. You're a great coach!"

Situation #4: The mother is in transition and she is sitting backward on the toilet. During contractions, she leans forward and relaxes. Once she is stable and ready, the coach says, "let it go" in a deeply relaxing tone as he rubs her back and encourages her. He reminds her to open up and relax under her abdomen and through her birth canal, so the baby can ease its way lower and lower. He encourages her to keep her hands loose and limp, and relaxed and to use slow and easy abdominal breathing. Her contractions are very powerful now, so he gives her constant encouragement and support. When the contraction is over, he gives her some praise and a sip of water (or juice, or whatever she is drinking).

Suggestions of ways the assistant coach might support this couple:
- Change the chux pad or towel on the bed so that when she returns, everything is clean and ready.
- Bring the coach a pillow that he can offer to the mother. (She might like something softer to lean over onto.)
- Bring the coach a step stool to sit on while he rubs her back. (Sitting on his knees may not be comfortable for long.)

- Be sure the mother is able to place each foot flat on the floor. If she is not, bring her two phone books (or whatever you can find) to place under each of her feet so they can rest flat.
- (She is likely to feel more supported this way and may avoid some additional stress and tension in the pelvis that can come from flexing her feet or resting on her toes.)
- Keep the sipper bottle filled.
- Answer the phone if it rings; keep their family and friends calm.
- If one of the medical professionals enters the room, say, **"Isn't she doing great!"**
- Tell her, **"You're doing fine. I believe in you!"**
- Tell him, **"You're amazing!"**

Situation #5: The mother is in first stage labor and has just returned to the bed from the bathroom. She needs to rest for a while. The coach helps her into the side relaxation position. He adjusts the pillows just the way she likes them with one that goes partly under her head and partly between her breasts, and another one or two under her top leg. He may also put a pillow under her top arm, behind her back and/or under her abdomen (whatever makes her most comfortable). As the next contraction begins, he says "relax, and let it go" in a deeply relaxing tone. As she exhales, you can see her body sink into the pillows and the bed. He strokes down her hair and across her shoulders. He continues stroking down her arms and all the way out her finger tips as he encourages her to relax down and out, down and through. The mother uses slow and easy abdominal breathing which naturally increases as the contractions reach their peak (at approximately 30 seconds). He massages her back, and then down her legs, and all the way out her toes. When the contraction is over, he gives her some well-deserved praise and a sip of water (or juice, or whatever she is drinking).

Suggestions of ways the assistant coach might support this couple:
- Check to be sure the bed is ready before she gets there. It should have a clean chux pad or towel on it and plenty of pillows. Be sure the sheets are turned down.
- Help the coach support her as she walks, if necessary.
- When she reaches the bed, offer to hold on to her for a moment so the coach can go around to the other side of the bed to assist her as she lays down.
- Get any extra pillows he may need for her.
- Go get her sipper bottle from the bathroom.
- Go get a hot water bottle if she would like one on her abdomen or lower back.
- Offer to turn on her favorite relaxing music.
- Keep the environment quiet and peaceful.
- Offer to turn the lights down.
- Get the coach something to eat and drink.
- Hand him the sipper bottle when the contraction is over.
- Offer to take over rubbing her back for a while so the coach can sit in front of her and hold her hand.
- Go in the other room and let them have some privacy.
- Tell her, "You're doing so well!"
- Tell him, "Good idea! She needs some rest."

Situation #6: The mother is in late first stage and just arriving at the birth place. She waits in the car until one more contraction is over, and then quickly gets out before the next contraction comes. The coach holds on to her and supports her as they slowly begin walking toward the door. While they are walking, she gets a contraction, so she stops. He comes around in front of her and puts his hands under her arms and around her back. He reminds her to stand with her feet wide apart so that she feels more stable, and her knees slightly bent to relieve pressure off her lower back. At about 10 seconds into the contraction, or whenever she is stable and he is ready, he says, "let it go". She responds by bending her knees and leaning forward into his arms so he can support more of her weight. He reminds her to relax, by closing her eyes, opening her mouth slightly, and relaxing her tongue. He asks her to release any tension around her shoulders and to relax down her arms making her open hands loose, limp, and relaxed. He lets her know every 15 seconds during the contraction. When the contraction is over, he asks her if she needs a boost up. If she does, he slowly counts to three and boosts her up to a standing position, then holds on to her while she gets her balance. He gives her praise, and a sip of water (or juice, or whatever she is drinking), and they continue walking into their birth place.

Suggestions of ways the assistant coach might support this couple:
- Carry her pillow(s), sipper bottle, bags, etc. for him.
- Close and lock the car. Be sure the coach has the key.
- Notice where the car is parked and if there are any time limits or restrictions on parking there.
- Help the coach support her as she walks, if necessary.
- If they have to stop in the middle of the street or parking lot for the contraction, stand beside them and signal cars to stop or go around them.
- Offer to go in and make the staff aware that they have arrived.
- Find out what room she will be in. While she and the coach slowly make their way in, you set up the room with her pillow(s), sipper bottle, music, etc. Set the temperature and the lighting so that it will be comfortable for her. When she gets to the room, it should be set up and ready for her.
- Answer any of the staff's questions so that the coach can keep his attention on her as much as possible.
- Communicate positively with the staff. Be friendly and polite.
- Give the coach a hand with anything he needs to do.
- Tell her, "I'm so proud of you!"
- Tell him, "You are very good at this!"
- Tell the staff, "this is such a great hospital (or birth center). That's why we came here!"

Situation #7: The mother is in second stage. She is in a side position, relaxing between contractions. The coach is wiping her brow with a cool wash cloth and encouraging her to close her eyes and rest between contractions. As the contraction begins, she takes a deep breath and then exhales it. She takes a second deep breath and exhales it. As she takes her third deep breath and holds it, she pulls her legs back, curls forward and puts her chin on her chest. The coach encourages her to "open up and push down and out". When she needs to, she leans her head back and exhales, then takes another deep breath. Then she puts her head down again, putting her chin on her chest, and continues pushing. The coach helps her rotate her head up to exhale, and down to push. She takes several breaths during each contraction. When the contraction is over, the coach gives her some well-earned praise, and a sip of water or some ice chips to suck on. He reminds her to relax completely as they wait for the next contraction to begin.

Suggestions of ways the assistant coach might support this couple:

♦ Stand behind the mother and help hold her legs up if necessary (during contractions her legs need to be pulled back toward her ears, not toward the ceiling. If she pulls her legs back rather than apart, there will be less stress on the perineum).
♦ Rinse the washcloth off to keep it cool and fresh.
♦ Get warm compresses for the mother's perineum, if you are asked to.
♦ Get any extra pillows he may need for her.
♦ Keep her sipper bottle or cup of ice chips filled.
♦ Stay out of the way of the medical professionals.
♦ Don't touch any sterile instruments or sterile drapes.
♦ Offer to take pictures.
♦ Be positive and encouraging.
♦ Hand him the sipper bottle or cup of ice chips when the contraction is over.
♦ Tell her, "Great job! It's getting closer and closer!"
♦ Tell him, "You are so good with her!"
♦ Tell the staff, "Don't they work well together?"

RESOURCES

The Bradley Method®-Student Workbook, by Marjie and Jay Hathaway, AAHCC, Susan Bek, AAHCC and James Hathaway, VP-AAHCC

Husband-Coached Childbirth by Robert A. Bradley, MD

Natural Childbirth the Bradley® Way, by Susan McCutcheon, AAHCC

Children At Birth, by Marjie and Jay Hathaway, AAHCC

Exercises for True Natural Childbirth, by Rhondda Hartman, AAHCC

What Every Pregnant Woman Should Know, By Gail Sforza Brewer and Tom Brewer, MD

The Birth Center, by Salee Berman, CNM, AAHCC and Victor Berman, MD. AAHCC

Emergency Childbirth, by Gregory White, MD

The Birth Book, By William Sears, MD and Martha Sears, RN

The Womanly Art of Breastfeeding, by La Leche League International

Nutrition Almanac, by Lavon J. Dunne

For further information about The Bradley Method®,
please contact:

www.bradleybirth.com

The Bradley Method® National Headquarters
Box 5224
Sherman Oaks, California 91413-5224
(800) 4-A-BIRTH
or
(818) 788-6662

GLOSSARY OF TERMS

LABOR AND BIRTH VOCABULARY

This glossary includes terms found in this book as well as many of the most common terms used in relation to labor and birth. You may find it helpful to become familiar with these terms in advance. Keep this book handy during labor so that you can quickly look up any terms you don't remember or understand. Do not be afraid to ask your medical professionals to explain anything to you that you don't understand.

AAHCC: American Academy of Husband-Coached Childbirth®; the organization that trains and certifies Bradley Method® instructors.

ABC: alternative birth center.

ACOG: American College of Obstetricians and Gynecologists

Abdominal breathing: moving air into and out of the lungs by movement of the diaphragm muscle, not the chest wall.

Afterbirth pains: contractions of the uterus after the birth is completed which help return the uterus to it's proper size, and reduce blood loss.

Afterbirth: the placenta and membranes expelled after the baby is born.

Amniotomy: artificially breaking the bag of waters.

Analgesia: a chemical or drug agent that reduces the perception of pain without loss of consciousness; narcotic; relaxer (sic).

Anemia: lower than normal amounts of red blood cells in the blood, sometimes called low blood count.

Anesthesia: a chemical or drug agent that causes loss of consciousness or complete cessation of pain reception, permitting surgery or other painful procedures.

Anterior presentation: presenting part of the baby is rotated so the occipital bone (back of the head) is toward the front of the mother; most common presentation.

Apgar rating: named for Dr. Virginia Apgar, a rating of the baby's condition immediately after birth, 2 points each for: heart rate, respiration, muscle tone, reflexes and color.

Areola: the darkened ring surrounding the nipple of the breast.

B.E.S.T.: Bradley® Energy-Saving Techniques

Bag of waters: the membranes that surround the baby and the amniotic fluid in the uterus; BOW; amnion is the inner layer, chorion is the outer layer.

Balanced diet: a harmonious portion of parts or elements in the diet. Supplying all essential and supplemental nutrients in their proper balance.

Birth canal: vagina.

Birth place: place where birth is planned to occur, or does occur. May be home, hospital, birth center or other place.

Birth plan: a written plan expressing the families desires in a normal birth, and also for possible complications.

Birth team: medical professionals, family, friends and support persons selected by the family to share the joy and enhance the comfort and safety of their birth.

Bloody show: passage of blood tinged mucous or mucous plug prior to onset of labor, or in labor. There is no fixed time before labor begins.

BOW: bag of waters.

BP: blood pressure.

Braxton-Hicks contractions: also called pre-labor or false-labor contractions; normal, common, intermittent, painless uterine contractions in the last six months of pregnancy.

Breech presentation: baby is coming foot, feet or buttocks first

Centimeter: a unit of length, approximately 2.5 centimeters per inch. One penny is 2 cm. is diameter.

Cervix: "baby door"; the neck of the uterus; the lower end of the uterus.

Cesarean section: surgical opening of abdomen and uterus to remove baby.

Chux pads: disposable underpads that laboring women often sit or lie on.

Circumcision: surgically removing the foreskin form a male baby's penis. Done for religious or personal reasons.

CNM: Certified Nurse Midwife

Colostrum: "Nature's vaccine for the newborn", American Academy of Pediatrics, fluid in the breast prior to the milk "coming in".

Complications: a variation from normal birth which carries an increased risk. Some are relatively minor (posterior or breech), some are major (prolapsed cord, hemorrhage).

Consumerism: an approach to childbearing wherein the parents take the active decision making role, with the active support and consultation of carefully selected medical professionals.

Contraction: shortening or tightening of a muscle, such as the uterus, once were called "pains".

Core temperature: temperature in the innermost part of the body, normal is 98.6 degrees Fahrenheit.

Crowning: the portion of second stage labor when the baby's head pushes the vulva forward looking like a crown.

Deficiency: absence of something essential; shortage; deficit.

Dehydration: excessive loss of water from the body.

Dilation: opening; the act of opening the cervix to approximately 10 cm.

Due date: an educated guess as to the expected date of birth.

Duration: how long a contraction lasts.

Effacement: thinning; the act of thinning the cervix, expressed in percentage.

EFM: electronic fetal monitoring.

Embryo: developing human baby the second through eighth week after conception.

Emergency childbirth: birth in other than the expected place, or with other than the expected people.

Emotional signpost: emotional state which helps predict the stage of labor the mother is in.

Engaged/dropped: the entrance of the presenting part of the baby into the pelvis prior to birth.

Episiotomy: surgical incision made in the perineum.

External version: turning the unborn baby by pressure through the mother's abdominal wall to alter the baby's position.

Fetal Heimlich maneuver: natural phenomenon, as baby is born mother's intact perineum pushes inward below the baby's rib-cage expelling mucous from baby's mouth and nose.

Fetoscope: a stethoscope used to listen to (auscultate) the baby's heart tones and other sounds.

Fetus: the unborn baby between the ninth week and birth.

Fontanel: normal soft spots or gaps in the skull of the baby.

Frequency: how often the contractions occur. Time from the beginning of one to the beginning of the next one.

Full term: truly ready to be born, usually 40-42 weeks after conception.

Gestation: growth of the baby from conception to birth while the mother supports and nourishes it.

Hawthorne effect: the effect of personal attention, seen in industrial engineering as well as in labor.

High risk: any condition of pregnancy which creates a higher than normal risk.

Hyperventilation: over-breathing leading to an abnormally low level of carbon dioxide (CO_2)

Hypothermia: too low a body temperature.

Hypovolemia: absence of normal increase, or abnormally decreased volume of circulating blood in the body.

Incubator: enclosed, heated, controlled holder for babies

Informed consent: the act of agreeing to a medical procedure after receiving information regarding it's benefits and risks, and weighing them and making up your own mind

Intensity: how strong contractions are.

Involution: return of the uterus to it's normal size and position after birth.

Ischial spines: bony prominences at lower edge of pelvis (narrowest part of pelvis), serves as measuring point of baby's decent, point called zero station.

IV: by intravenous injection.

Jaundice: hyperbilirubinemia; a yellowing of the skin and/or whites of the eyes.

Kegel: either a name for the pelvic floor muscle (pubococcygeous), or exercises to strengthen it, or the man who discovered it (Dr. Arnold Kegel)

Labor coach: husband or other supportive person selected by mother to assist in preparation for and the act of birthing.

Labor Support Professional: LSP; a person who is specially trained to provide additional physical and emotional support to couples in labor

Lactation: breastfeeding; the function of secreting milk.

LDR: labor, delivery, recovery—a multipurpose hospital room.

LLL: La Leche League; a group of experienced mothers who help and support good mothering through breastfeeding.

LOA: left occiput anterior.

Local anesthetic: an injection of a narcotic in the skin which will soon spread to the whole body and the baby. "There is no such thing as a *local*", Dr. Bradley.

Lochia: the bloody discharge for several weeks following birth.

Low risk: a normal pregnancy, may have many variations but remains within a normal risk range.

LSP: Labor Support Professional

Malar flush: a reddish color of the cheeks, typical of the onset of labor . . . but not always.

Meconium staining: appearance of bowel movement from the baby in the amniotic fluid prior to birth, a fairly common occurrence. Most often normal, but may indicate distress.

Meconium: black, sticky, tarry substance excreted during baby's first bowel movements. Can continue for three days then changes to normal newborn bowel movement.

Medication: a drug, chemical or other agent used to relieve pain or treat disease.

Modesty: not displaying one's body—a condition which gradually disappears during labor.

Motivation: motivation, or being motivated; to give impetus to; to incite; to impel.

Moulding: the shaping of the baby's head to the shape and size of the birth canal.

Mucous plug: a blob of mucous passed by the mother as the cervix begins to dilate. May be well before the onset of labor.

Multigravida: a woman who has been pregnant two or more times.

Multipara: a woman who has given birth to two or more babies.

Natural alignment plateau: NAP; the normal period in many labors when dilation is not increasing, but uterine activity continues. Often ends with rapid complete dilation.

Natural childbirth: as your great-great grandmother have birth; childbirth regarded and performed as a natural process without analgesia, anesthesia or surgery.

Neonatal: pertaining to a newborn baby.

NPO: from the Latin "non per os"—nothing by mouth; withholding of food and liquid.

Nursery: the department in a hospital where newborn babies are cared for.

Nutrients: essential substances which affect the metabolic and growth processes in the mother or the baby.

OB: Obstetrician

OB/GYN: Obstetrician/Gynecologist

OP: occiput posterior; baby's occipital bone (back of the head) toward mother's back; "sunny-side up". Causes "back labor".

PA-C: Physicians Assistant-Certified

Parturition: the act of birthing.

PE: pressure episiotomy.

Pediatrician: a doctor who specializes in dealing with children.

Pelvic floor: supportive muscle surrounding the urethra, vagina and rectum, extends from symphysis pubis in front to coccyx in back.

Pelvis: basin-like ring of bone at the bottom of the mother's spine through which the baby must pass to be born.

Perineal massage: massaging the perineum, either during pregnancy or in labor. It's purpose is to thin the perineum, and add to it's elasticity. It may reduce the chance of tearing or needing an episiotomy.

Perineum: the skin and muscles between the vagina and the anus.

Physiological pushing: positive pushing; mother-initiated pushing, only to the point of comfort, holding breath only as long as comfortable, tuning-in to her own body's instructions and urges.

Pica: a craving for unusual foods during pregnancy.

PKU: phenylketonuria; either a test or the name of a disease (indicating inborn error of metabolism) where baby is unable to digest phenylalanine, can lead to retardation. Very rare (approximately one in 40,000).

Placenta: the afterbirth; organ grown from outer layer of the egg which grows to nourish the baby. Mother's blood and baby's blood circulate within the placenta and transfer oxygen, nutrients and wastes but their bloods do not mix.

Positive communications: being able to express your preferences and decisions in such a way as to retain the enthusiastic support of your birth team.

The Bradley Method® *ASSISTANT COACH'S MANUAL*

Positive pain: pain with a purpose, whose meaning is to inform you of progress, needed changes, etc.

Posterior presentation: baby's occipital bone (back of the head) is toward the mothers spine. Causes "back labor".

Postmature baby: often merely means an error in estimating due date, or a pregnancy that really is longer than average. In true postmaturity, means a seriously ill baby; placenta or mother are not supplying needed nutrients, baby's skin is falling loose, baby losing weight, subcutaneous fat layer is gone, baby looks like a very old dying person. Very rare event

Postpartum: the period after a baby is born.

Pre labor: before labor.

Pre-eclampsia: also called toxemia; those symptoms often believed to be predictive of eclampsia; edema, proteinuria and hypertension.

Premature baby: a baby born before it is mature enough to thrive without assistance, not necessarily related to weight alone.

Prep: procedures done by the medical staff to prepare mother for delivery, may include: shave, enema, blood pressure measurement, blood sample, urine sample, vaginal exam(s), fetal monitor strip, history, etc.

Pressure episiotomy: PE; episiotomy performed without narcotics, birth attendant waits until crowning, cuts during a contraction when the stretched perineum is without circulation and sensation is naturally reduced.

Primigravida: a woman during her first pregnancy.

Primipara: a woman who has had one baby.

PROM: premature rupture of membranes.

Protein: organic substances essential in the diet, containing amino acids; primary substances for human life and growth.

Pubic bone: symphysis pubis; the front portion of the pelvis.

Pubococcygeous muscle: also called the PC muscle, the pelvic floor muscle, supports abdominal organs and uterus (see Kegel).

Realistic expectations: recognizing the inherent risk of childbearing and the irreducible hazards. Alsobeing realistic about what kind of support you can expect to receive from the birth team and birth place you have chosen. Accepting the normal variations in labor and birth regarding time, work, and pain.

Recovery: often used to describe the immediate period after a birth, surgery or procedure.

Rectum: portion of large intestine connection to the anus.

Respiratory depression: lower than normal frequency or depth of respiration.

RN: Registered Nurse

Sitz baths: shallow water bath

Stamina: resistance to fatigue; endurance; staying power.

Station: the downward progress of the baby relative to the ischial spines, expressed in centimeters i.e.: -1, +2, etc.

Supine position: lying flat on your back.

Third stage: expulsion of the placenta

Toxemia: also called pre-eclampsia, life-threatening disease of pregnancy leading to eclampsia (convulsions).

Transition: the change from first stage labor to second stage, often a short but stressful time marked by confusion.

Transverse lie: a baby lying sideways in the uterus, if the mother is in active labor this is a true complication. Very rare.

Trimester: one-third portion of pregnancy, about three months.

Umbilical cord: connects the baby to it's placenta. Contains two arteries and one vein. Is also a part of the endocrine system, manufactures hormones.

Urethra: tube that carries urine from the bladder to exterior of the body.

Urge to push: signals from mother or baby's body to mother that additional effort is needed to expel baby or to align uterus by the mother's own efforts.

Uterus: "baby box"; hollow muscular organ in which the baby grows and is nourished, also called the womb.

Vaginal Exam: entering the vagina, usually with a gloved finger or hand, to access the dilation, effacement, station, and presentation. May increase the risk of infection. (see Student Workbook page 42)

The Bradley Method® *ASSISTANT COACH'S MANUAL*

VBAC: vaginal birth after cesarean

Vernix caseosa: "baby cold cream"; white, cheesy substance which protects the baby's skin in the uterus. It also moisturizes the baby's skin when rubbed in after birth.

Vertex presentation: head down, baby's head is positioned to come through the pelvis ahead of the rest of the body.